THE
ENHANCED SERVICES
HANDBOOK

Commissioning Editor: Alison Taylor

Development Editor: Catherine Jackson

Project Manager: Rachel Wheeler

Production Manager: Andy Hannan

Design and Typesetting: The Designers Collective Limited

THE ENHANCED SERVICES HANDBOOK

Andrew Dearden MBBCh, MRCGP

Principal GP, Cardiff;

Chairman, GPC Wales;

Member, UK GPC Negotiating Team;

Chairman, BMA Pensions Committee

Foreword by

Hamish Meldrum BSc, MBChB, DRCOG, FRCGP

Chairman, GPC, British Medical Association

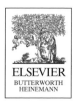

ELSEVIER
BUTTERWORTH
HEINEMANN

Edinburgh London New York Oxford
Philadelphia St Louis Sydney Toronto 2006

ELSEVIER
BUTTERWORTH
HEINEMANN

First published 2006

ISBN 0 7506 8891 2

British Library Cataloguing in Publication Data
A catalogue record for this book is available from the British Library

Library of Congress Cataloging in Publication Data
A catalogue record for this book is available from the Library of Congress

Notice
Knowledge and best practice in this field are constantly changing. As new research and experience broaden our knowledge, changes in practice, treatment and drug therapy may become necessary or appropriate. Readers are advised to check the most current information provided (i) on procedures featured or (ii) by the manufacturer of each product to be administered, to verify the recommended dose or formula, the method and duration of administration, and contraindications. It is the responsibility of the practitioner, relying on their own experience and knowledge of the patient, to make diagnoses, to determine dosages and the best treatment for each individual patient, and to take all appropriate safety precautions. To the fullest extent of the law, neither the publisher nor the author assumes any liability for any injury and/or damage.

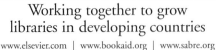

Working together to grow
libraries in developing countries

www.elsevier.com | www.bookaid.org | www.sabre.org

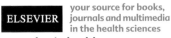

ELSEVIER   BOOK AID
            International   Sabre Foundation

ELSEVIER   your source for books,
            journals and multimedia
            in the health sciences
www.elsevierhealth.com

The
Publisher's
policy is to use
**paper manufactured
from sustainable forests**

Printed in China

Dedication

To my Mum and Dad, Wendy and Phil.

Many agree that how a person does in a race depends to a great extent to the quality of their start. I would say the same of life, and I could not have had a better one.
Truly 'goodly parents'.

Acknowledgements

To all those have worked tirelessly in trying to get enhanced services up and running in their area. All I can say is that it does get easier, and it is worth it in the end!

Thanks to *Doctor* magazine for allowing me to include a previously published article in Chapter 8 on 'How to say no'.

My thanks to the numerous GPs, local medical committees, primary care trusts and local health boards for giving me permission to include their worked-up examples of enhanced services in this book.

My thanks to the members and staff of the General Practitioners Committee (GPC) for their long and hard work in the area of enhanced services, some of which is included here. Special thanks to all the staff of the GPC who worked on the various guidance notes referred to here and to Justin Cross for the use of his summary of negotiating principles.

Contents

Foreword

As Andrew Dearden indicates, enhanced services have been described as one of the most contentious and exasperating areas of the new general medical services (GMS) contract. However, despite this they remain a crucial feature of the contract's ability to help control GP workload by giving practices the opportunity to say 'no' to unresourced work. In many ways, I prefer to think of them as a much more positive opportunity; one where practices can be enabled to say 'yes', but with the crucial provisos that they wish to take on new work and the resources are there for them to do it.

As with any system, there have been very significant teething problems, with both primary care organisations (PCOs) and practices trying to draw their own, very different, lines in the sand. However, where they have worked well – and there are many examples of this – enhanced services have shown how they can be used to tailor effective local services for patients. I hope that over time they will become a vehicle that will allow an appropriate shift from secondary to primary care so that patients can have better, local access to key services.

Andrew has used his experience both as a negotiator and an advisor to many local medical committees (LMCs), to produce a book that will be an invaluable tool for practices and LMCs directly involved in the discussions and negotiations around the delivery of enhanced services. It should also be required reading for PCO managers! Not only does it describe the thinking that led to the development of enhanced services, it gives detailed and practical advice to help develop service specifications and determine pricing.

There are useful chapters on negotiating skills and examples of established enhanced services, together with detailed appendices giving fully worked specifications, including pricing.

As some wag observed, in the NHS the status quo is always changing. Enhanced services can help to ensure that changes take place in a way that allows practices to choose to take on new work safely and appropriately for both practices and patients alike. Andrew Dearden's short but comprehensive book will greatly help that process.

Hamish Meldrum
Chairman, General Practitioners Committee
British Medical Association

Introduction

Enhanced services have been called both one of the most welcome, and one of the most frustrating parts of the new GMS contract. Many GPs can see the benefits of the concept and are anxious to be able to provide enhanced services for their patients, but they feel frustrated at the lack of progress in their area. In some parts of the UK, PCOs have caught the vision of enhanced services and their potential to improve patient care, especially for those most vulnerable in society. But where GPs and LMCs are struggling, they find that even after a huge amount of preparation and extended discussions with their PCO, they keep running into brick walls when it comes to actually agreeing and establishing enhanced services. I hope this will become a less frequent occurrence, but I feel that until the issue of secondary care 'debt' or overspend is properly dealt with, the competing priorities for new money will continue to inhibit service developments.

In this book I want to try to help as much as possible with the work needed to prepare a business case and submission for an enhanced service to your PCO. I will cover areas like what can be defined as an enhanced service, what can be included and what can't, how to put together a business plan or proposal, costs to remember when doing so and how to say 'no' to unresourced, unpaid work.

I have been involved in negotiating local development schemes (LDSs) and now enhanced services for the past eight years. I have to say that the first few years of trying to get LDSs off the ground was like pulling teeth, with quite a lot of forceful discussions involved. So I can fully understand the frustration felt by those at the beginning of the process. What I have found is that once PCOs start to use enhanced services to provide care they find they get a better service at a more cost-effective price. This, I think, leads them to see the advantages of enhanced services and the process does get easier.

CHAPTER 1
WHY ENHANCED SERVICES?

One of the major points that came from the series of GP surveys carried out before the new contract negotiations, was the need for GPs to be able to control their workload. This came up again and again and was always at the top of the list of issues that needed to be addressed in the negotiations. GPs made it quite clear in their responses to these surveys that workload was one of the greatest problems faced by general practice in terms of both recruitment to the profession and retention of the current workforce. Many GPs stated that they felt the workload was unsustainable and would lead them to reduce their commitment to the NHS or to leave the NHS entirely, either by career shift or early retirement.

The old contract's 'Red Book' had what was affectionately called the 'John Wayne clause' because it could be summarised as 'a GP's gotta do, what a GP's gotta do!' I am told that this quote is wrongly attributed to John Wayne, but you know what I mean! Basically, the Red Book seemed to suggest that we had to see everyone and anyone who walked through our door, and that we had almost no ability to say 'no' to work we didn't want to do. This included any work that the secondary care sector suddenly decided it was no longer going to provide and so had to be done by GPs. It did not matter that we may not have had the staff or resources to provide the care required or, more worryingly, that we may not have had the clinical skills and training to provide the service needed; we seemed to have no choice.

This had to change. It began to change with the introduction of the core/non-core strategy by the former General Medical Services Committee, now called the General Practitioners Committee (GPC). It was formalised into enhanced services during the new contract negotiations.

But I feel some of us have lost sight of the reasons why we wanted classification or categorisation of services, like enhanced services, in the first place. We wanted it and needed it to control our workload, so we could say 'no' to work that we didn't want to do or were unable to provide because of lack of resources, skills, etc. Before the new contract we said that the workload was 'killing us'. Oddly enough, some of us now seem to say 'pay us enough and we'll kill ourselves'! Enhanced services were not just about getting paid; they were about gaining the ability and the confidence to say 'no' as well. We need to remember that the principle of enhanced services gives us the ability to do both.

This was made very clear in paragraph 3.16 (one of my very favourite paragraphs!) of the new contract documentation in the original 'Blue Book'.

"There will be no obligation on practices to provide any enhanced service (notwithstanding that they have previously provided it) unless they enter into a new contract for its provision."

This means that even if you have been providing a service that is now classified as an enhanced service (e.g. INR monitoring), whether you have been paid for it or not, you will be under no obligation to continue the service unless you enter into a new contract. If the PCO refuses to offer you a new contract, you are fully within your rights to inform the PCO of your intention to withdraw from this enhanced service.

So, enhanced services had two main purposes:

- To get paid for work we were already doing or wanted to be able to provide. It created a payment structure we could use to agree payment and PCOs could use to develop services for patients
- To be able to classify a new service (or an old service someone was trying to dump on us) in such a way that GPs could, with contractual protection, decline to provide such a service.

I feel we are focusing so much on the first purpose that we may have forgotten the second. I think that in a few years we will look back and see that the concept of enhanced services benefited us most not by the money it brought into practices, but by the unwanted, unresourced work we were able to decline.

Now, that said, many GPs and LMCs are getting much more confident at saying 'no' to unresourced work. Many now feel they have contractual backing to be able to do so, which they do in fact have. It is vital that we remember that within practices, areas and nationally we have the right to say 'no' to work that is not part of essential services. Even knowing and remembering this can increase our confidence when we negotiate with our PCO.

CHAPTER 2
ENHANCED SERVICES WITHIN THE NEW GMS CONTRACT

In a letter to the Local Health Boards (LHBs) (the equivalent of primary care trusts [PCTs] in Wales) in October 2003, the Welsh Assembly Government listed what it saw as the purpose and objectives of enhanced services. It said:

"The key objectives of enhanced services are to:
- *Improve patient care for all patients and for specific vulnerable groups*
- *Allow practices to develop services for their practice populations*
- *Improve patient choice*
  Aid the shift of work from secondary care to primary care."

If you add allowing GPs to say 'no' to unwanted or unresourced, unfunded work, I think this is a pretty good summary of what enhanced services can be used to achieve.

The new contract framework document published in April 2002 outlined the plans to include a classification of services called 'enhanced services'. These plans were a natural development of the LDSs that came out of the non-core document produced by the General Medical Services Committee in 1996.

There are three types of enhanced services:
- Directed
- National
- Local.

Directed enhanced services

A directed enhanced service (DES) is an enhanced scheme that your PCO is obligated to provide. The PCO has no option because it is legally obliged to provide these services in its area. **Box 1** lists the six schemes designated as DESs.

These should now be in place. Details can be found in the *GMS Statement of Financial Entitlement* (available at www.dh.gov.uk). The

---

BOX 1   DIRECTED ENHANCED SERVICES

1. Minor surgery
2. Violence
3. Influenza immunisation
4. Access
5. Childhood vaccinations and immunisations
6. Preparation of records for quality (summarising notes)

---

sixth DES – preparation of records for quality – is time limited and ran only for the first two years of the new contract, i.e. 2003/4 and 2004/5.

National enhanced services

National enhanced services (NESs) were services for which it was possible to agree general specifications and pricing structures at national level during the negotiations on the new contract. We wanted to have a set of enhanced services that many GPs were already providing or wanted to be able to provide in their surgeries. As such, we tried to pick those we felt would cover as many GPs' initial aspirations as possible.

In the very first contract framework document we suggested a num-

---

BOX 2   NATIONAL ENHANCED SERVICES

1. Anticoagulant monitoring
2. Shared-care drug monitoring
3. Depression
4. Alcohol misuse
5. Insertion of intrauterine devices
6. Drug misuse
7. Multiple sclerosis
8. Immediate care
9. Minor injuries
10. Sexual health

ber of NESs. They included the 10 listed in **Box 2** and two others: nursing homes and learning difficulties. These two did not make it into the final group of NESs for various reasons (ask me about it sometime), but have now been commissioned in many areas of the UK. It is fair to say that the GPC negotiating team was very keen to include these two, especially nursing homes because it was a major area of workload shift and perfect for an enhanced service.

Although the list of NESs had been agreed as part of the negotiations, many local discussions have modified them to better suit individual arrangements and preferences. This is totally up to local GPs, practices and LMCs. It may be appropriate to change the specification to suit local circumstances, but the PCO should not use this to try to reduce the price while keeping the work the same. We must not accept any diminution of the price, without a corresponding reduction in the work expected. Where appropriate, the NESs might be seen as a 'starter for 10'. They can be updated also in terms of clinical practices or service specifications. As with all clinical or medical services, they are meant to evolve and develop in line with recognised good practice.

Specifications and pricing for the NESs listed in Box 2 are given in the supporting documentation of the new contract.

Local enhanced services

This is definitely the most wide ranging group. GPs, LMCs and PCOs have worked together in many areas to establish a range of local enhanced services (LESs). A recent GPC advice note (Appendix 1) on enhanced services listed a range of LESs already set up and being paid for as enhanced services. This long list includes:
- All the DESs and NESs
- Nursing homes/residential homes
- Asylum seekers
- Prescribing and monitoring lithium
- Prescribing and monitoring drugs not mentioned in the 'near-patient testing' NES. This includes amiodarone, gold and sulphasalazine
- Initiation of secondary care drugs. This includes insulin and initial monitoring under shared-care agreements, such as depot psychotropics, methylphenidate and prescribing for alcohol dependency
- Suture removal
- Dressings post operation/leg ulcers
- Minor/moderate surgery. This includes vasectomy, sigmoidoscopy, carpal tunnel release and in-growing toenails
- GP with a special interest (GPwSI) working in the community. If the

GPwSI is working in the community and providing enhanced community GMS, this can count towards the enhanced services floor (see Chapter 3). In addition, to count towards the floor, the referral pathway should be GP to GPwSI and not via secondary care. This includes dermatology, psychosexual counselling, allergy, genetic counselling, joint injections, vasectomy, cystoscopy, heart failure, gynaecology and podiatry

- Goserelin/finasteride/oestrogen/etonogestrel-releasing contraceptive implants. These implants are not and have never been part of ordinary primary medical services and they need special training and techniques
- Depo-Provera contraceptive implants
- Collecting information for PCOs. This includes validating waiting lists
- Immunisations not otherwise covered in essential or additional services. This includes giving MMR to students and hepatitis B for occupational health reasons
- Evening/weekend surgeries if done by practices at the PCO's request and funded by the PCO. This does not include emergency work
- More specialised chronic disease care schemes (GPwSI type)
- Pre-operative assessments requested by the hospital. This includes MRSA screening
- Medical certificates for patients who have been in hospital
- Phlebotomy that is not an essential part of GMS. This includes blood tests as requested by the hospital and/or outpatients' department
- 24-Hour blood pressure monitoring
- Cardiac event monitoring
- Neonatal checks
- Audiology screening
- Glaucoma screening
- Teenage sexual health drop-in clinics
- Obesity/weight management services
- Counselling. This includes contestable services provided by an independent organisation in the community and available to all the GP's patients and/or provided within surgeries
- ECGs at the hospital's request. This does not include routine ECGs for hypertension, palpitations or chest pain
- Unscheduled vaccinations.

The GPC advice note also contained a list of services that should not be classified as enhanced services. This included:
- GPwSI working in hospitals. If a GPwSI is working as a clinical assistant or staff grade in a routine outpatient clinic, this cannot count

towards the enhanced services floor, which includes a GPwSI service based in the community

- Therapies, such as physiotherapy
- Pharmacy work, such as pharmacy advisers
- Dental work
- Secondary care carried out in the community, such as work done by consultants and specialist nurses
- Community hospital current contacts (e.g. a new minor injury unit might count as an LES)
- Normal out-of-hours work
- Prescribing incentive schemes. These are not medical or patient services; they are not contestable; they are not provided for patients and the schemes have never been funded by GMS money (or hospital money), but from completely separate prescribing budgets
- Health promotion hosted services. This is standard health promotion activity and so is not an enhanced service, which the PCT hosts for the locality
- PRIMIS facilitator
- Citizens Advice workers (practice based). This is a social service rather than a clinical service, and it does not constitute providing patient care
- Evercare nursing model
- Medical certificates for patients who have been in hospital.

CHAPTER 3

THE ENHANCED SERVICE FLOOR: WHEN IS A FLOOR A CEILING?

The concept of the 'floor' came about during negotiations on the new contract. The GPC wanted to make sure it did not agree anything that became so deprived of funding that in effect nothing happened or no new patient services were provided. So the government decided to introduce the idea of a spending floor. This was meant to be a minimum amount (hence a floor) that PCOs would have to spend, and be expected to spend in their areas, on enhanced services each year. I still think the idea itself was sound, but with so many of these things it went a bit wonky during implementation.

The first problem in England was that although £350 million was allocated to PCOs for the enhanced services in the first year, rather than that money being 'new and additional' the government announced late in the process that the amount had been included in the financial allocations to PCTs at the start of the year, some months before. To be fair to the PCTs, this left them struggling to find money for new initiatives because the money 'allocated' for enhanced services had already been spent or allocated to other services. GPs and LMCs became increasingly frustrated when PCTs were initially reluctant to start talks on developing enhanced services.

In Wales it was approached in a different way. The money that made up the enhanced service floor allocation was kept at Welsh Assembly level and sent down to LHBs only after agreements had been reached at national level between the Welsh Assembly Government and GPC Wales. This has had the effect of making fairly sure that all the money has been spent in truly enhanced services and that most, if not all, of the money has been used to commission services from GP practices. We have been fortunate in Wales not to have seen the creative counting and accounting demonstrated by some PCTs when saying where the enhanced service money has been spent. We have been fairly reassured in Wales that most, if not all, of the enhanced services money has made its way to GPs, or at least it will have by April 2006.

The GPC guidance *Focus on Enhanced Services* (March 2005) on LMC involvement with establishing and agreeing the floor states:

"The LMC should be consulted about the proposed level of spend and the PCO should seek to obtain LMC agreement that the proposed services count within the above definition for financial monitoring purposes. Where there is a dispute over what counts towards the floor, the LMC and PCO should seek to resolve this locally in the first instance.

PCOs will be under a legal obligation to commission services for violent patients (from 1 February 2004), influenza immunisations, and minor surgery (both from 1 April 2004). These can be commissioned from any provider, or the PCO can provide the service itself. However, it is likely that PCOs will in most instances want to commission these services from the patients' own GMS and personal medical services (PMS) contractors, to ensure continuity of care."

Any problems that cannot be sorted out locally should be referred in the first instance to the enhanced services subgroup of the GPC's primary care development subcommittee.

CHAPTER 4
WHAT CAN BE CLASSIFIED AS AN ENHANCED SERVICE?

So how can you tell what can be classified as an enhanced service? What can be counted and what cannot be counted as an enhanced service seems to have confused many people. The definition used in the new contract documents is clear in some ways, but can be quite broad in others. The new contract guidance document Investing in Primary Care states in paragraphs 2.77 and 2.78:

"PCTs will be placed under a duty through directions to commission all six current Directed Enhanced Services (DES) to meet the needs of their population. In line with paragraph 2.13 of Investing in General Practice, the Contract Regulations define enhanced services as follows: 'medical services other than essential services, additional services or out of hours services; or essential services, additional services or out of hours services or an element of such a service that a contractor agrees under the contract to provide in accordance with specifications set out in a plan, which requires of the contractor an enhanced level of service provision to that which it needs generally to provide in relation to that service or element of service'. The Contract Regulations allow the medical services to be of any type, in any setting, and to extend beyond the scope of primary medical services. There is no legal constraint as to what types of NHS medical services a PCT can commission through the four provider routes described in section A of this chapter. This will give PCTs a broad ability to develop more integrated services across the primary, secondary and acute sectors.

"However, for the purposes of financial monitoring, the definition of enhanced services is drawn more tightly than the legal definition. PCTs will be notified of their enhanced services expenditure floor level in the January 2004 allocations, which

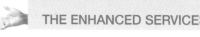

they will be expected to meet but can exceed. PCTs will need to consider carefully what constitutes an enhanced service for the purpose of accurate financial monitoring. This will be undertaken at national level by the joint BMA/NHS Confederation/Health Departments Technical Steering Committee. Whilst a precise national definition would not be sufficiently sensitive to local issues, PCTs and contractors should bear in mind that, generally speaking, the following spend would count towards the floor:

(i)   Commissioning, or direct PCT provision, of Directed, National or Locally Enhanced Services from any provider, not just GMS and PMS contractors

(ii) Practitioners With a Special Interest (PWSIs) except in relation to essential or additional services

(iii) The plus element of PMS Plus and the specialist element of specialist PMS arrangements

(iv) Local primary medical care incentive schemes commissioned from GMS or PMS providers

(v) If the PCT proposed, for example, to re-commission a service that had previously been placed with a NHS trust it would count towards the floor, regardless of the outcome of the contest, but only providing that:

  (a) It was contestable for GMS and PMS contractors

  (b) It is a service that might reasonably be provided by GMS and PMS contractors, for example because looking across the UK there are other such contractors delivering similar services."

This leads us to two simple sets of questions to ask of any proposed enhanced service to determine whether that particular service can be seen and funded as an enhanced service.

The first set should always produce the answer 'yes'. If the answer to any of these questions is 'no', then the proposed service probably would not count as an enhanced service.

- Does it provide a higher level or specialisation of care to patients?
- Is it contestable by GPs?
- Can it reasonably be provided by GPs?

The second set of questions should always produce the answer 'no'. A 'yes' answer to any of these questions would call into doubt the validity of the proposed service being an enhanced service.

- Is it spend on primary care services funded through other routes?
- Is it spend on essential services, e.g. premises, greenfield sites?
- Is it funding the provision of out-of-hours services?
- Is it baseline spend for services provided by trusts, e.g. accident and emergency services, existing services provided by GPs in community hospitals or as clinical assistants, and provided under an existing contract?
- Does it provide essential or additional services for patients?

CHAPTER 5

ARE GPs PREFERRED PROVIDERS FOR ENHANCED SERVICES?

A question that the GPC negotiators used to get asked a lot was 'are GPs preferred providers of enhanced services?'. We are still asked this occasionally, so I thought I'd include a brief chapter on the question.

GPs do have preferred provider status for the provision of additional services. These are the services that include cervical smears, childhood immunisations, maternity services, etc. However, we do not have preferred provider status for enhanced services (except for access and Quality and Incentives in Practice [QuIP], which are GP practice issues). This, hopefully, is not a shock to most of us because the new contract documents have always made this clear.

But many of us will already be providing some of these services. The contract documentation is quite clear: if you had an existing contract to provide these services (e.g. to provide a service for violent patients or INR monitoring) the existing contract should have continued after 1 April 2004 for at least the time agreed in the contract (see paragraph 2.15 (ii) in the new contract document). Of course, any contract can be ended by either party after a period of notice, or it can be renegotiated if both sides agree. This has always been the case and is not new or specific to the new contract.

But if a PCO decides to decommission a service from GPs it must then commission it from someone else. If you find yourself in this situation you must make absolutely sure that the PCT knows that you will then refer all patients who came under that particular enhanced service to the new provider. The PCO must not mistakenly believe that you will carry on doing the work even if you are not being paid for it.

It is theoretically possible for the PCO to use a provider outside GP practices but, in my opinion, it is practically impossible to find a provider that could do the job as effectively and in as patient friendly a way as we can. My reasons for thinking this? Look at what they have to replace if we are not involved:

- We provide services close to our patients
- We don't need to use hospital transport systems (although we might like to be able to!)

- We can identify at-risk populations relatively easily
- We see many of our patients regularly
- We already have the staff, premises and equipment for many services in place.

If a PCO were to undermine this proven system in the pursuit of what it thinks might be initial savings, it would be very unwise indeed. But remember that one of the main aims of the new contract was to decrease workload. That was the main concern GPs expressed in the various surveys undertaken before the start of the negotiations. It's not just about getting more money; it is about controlling our workload and stopping the work we don't want to do, as well as being paid for work we are willing to do.

If you do lose an enhanced service or don't get one started, remember that the quality and outcomes framework of the contract is the main source of substantial new funding. You can now afford to give up or stop some work because the money from the quality and outcomes framework will more than make up for the vast majority of enhanced service losses.

CHAPTER 6
HOW TO DEVELOP A SERVICE SPECIFICATION FOR ENHANCED SERVICES

When you or others have identified a need that could be met with an enhanced service, you will need to develop a service specification. This clearly outlines what you will provide and the contractual arrangements for provision and payment, and covers things like dispute resolution, audits, etc.

In the past we have done things on ad hoc arrangements where we got a sum of money (if we were lucky) and then just kind of got on with it. In these days of clinical governance and with an increasing culture of blame, it is vital that you have a service specification that makes it clear what is being commissioned and provided. Although some see this as a restriction, I would say it protects GPs and their staff.

I will cover all the areas I think you should have at least thought about, although it may not be necessary to include every area in every LES specification (see also Appendix 5). I have also included several actual enhanced service specifications in Appendices 9–19. I have used the Welsh gonadorelins enhanced service (Appendix 15) here to illustrate the relevant points.

Model LES for administration of gonadorelins

Introduction

For your introduction, you could include a paragraph such as:

"All practices are expected to provide essential and those additional services they are contracted to supply to all their patients. This specification outlines the more specialised services to be offered. The specification of this service is designed to cover enhanced aspects of clinical care of the patient that go beyond the scope of essential services. No part of the specification by commission, omission or implication defines or redefines essential or additional services."

Background

Many enhanced service specifications include an element of background to put the service being commissioned in context. In terms of the actual contract between two sides this is not always necessary, but it can often help others see why patients need this service. It can help outside people see why the service is being provided and what is actually being provided.

For example, an enhanced service for goserelin (Zoladex) might include the following paragraphs:

"Gonadorelins are used primarily, although not exclusively, for treating carcinoma of the prostate. There are a number of treatment regimes, which vary in the detail of their programme of administration and main purpose. Broadly they can be divided on the basis of the progress of the disease into advanced local disease and metastatic disease. The central use, however, is the treatment of metastatic cancer of the prostate. Currently, it is estimated that over 95% of the prescriptions for gonadorelin analogues are written for carcinoma of the prostate.

Virtually all the prescriptions issued for injectable gonadorelins are written by GPs and most of these are also administered by GPs. In some practices an appropriately trained practice nurse will site the depot implants. The great majority of prescriptions are issued for Zoladex (generic name goserelin), which is administered subcutaneously into the anterior abdominal wall as a depot implant. Others are given subcutaneously or intramuscularly, depending on the indications and the preparation.

There are several preparations (injectable and implants) for treating carcinoma of the prostate. These include: buserelin, goserelin, leuprorelin acetate and triptorelin. The most commonly used preparations for treating carcinoma of the prostate are goserelin implants or leuprorelin injections.

There are varying treatment models for administering gonadorelins to patients with carcinoma of the prostate, dependent on the clinical management programme agreed for that patient."

Patient groups covered by the service specification

It is always helpful to be absolutely clear about who and what is covered under the service specification. This will help ensure you meet each side's expectations and avoid ill feelings. The specification should also cover the timescale of the agreement with rollover arrangements. The model specification for administering gonadorelins included the following paragraphs:

"This model service has been agreed between the Welsh Assembly Government and the GPC (Wales) for the administration of gonadorelins for patients with prostate cancer only.

LHBs should commission this from April 2005 and may wish to use the uplift in the enhanced services allocations for 2005/6 to meet the costs."

Aims

Some specifications include general aims to help inform those not so closely associated with the work involved. This is not always needed but is often included for completeness. The model specification for administering gonadorelins included the following paragraphs:

"The administration of gonadorelins within primary care is designed to be an enhanced service in which:

Patients with an established diagnosis and agreed treatment plan of carcinoma of the prostate can undergo part of their treatment safely, effectively and conveniently close to their home.

There is much greater integration of primary and secondary care services and which recognises the increasing contribution that primary care can make in medical management and treatment of the hitherto predominantly hospital-based approach."

Service outline

This is where the real details are outlined and, as we know, 'the devil is in the detail'. It is here that much of the negotiation will take place. The higher the level of demand or work involved in the service being commissioned, the greater the resources needed to provide it. In my experience this is where the commissioners want everything but seemingly are prepared only to pay for some things. It is here you must concentrate your effort to ensure the service is safe for patients and attractive to GPs who might want to provide the service themselves.

The model specification for administering gonadorelins included the following paragraphs:

"It is a requirement of this national enhanced service that the contractor:

i. *Provides a register – practices will need to produce and maintain a valid up-to-date register of patients being treated as part of this enhanced service*

ii. *Demonstrates a call and recall system – practices will need to ensure a systematic call and recall of patients on this register is taking place, and have in place the means to identify and follow up patients in default*

iii. *Agrees a joint clinical management programme – patients should be managed on the basis of individual treatment plans, which will normally be drawn up by local consultants. Practices will be expected to follow these treatment plans unless there has been discussion and agreement with local consultants to modify them*

iv. *Supports the education of both newly diagnosed patients and those with established disease. The secondary care oncology team will provide the main source of advice for both newly diagnosed patients and those with established disease. The practice will reinforce and supplement that advice where appropriate to do so*

v. *Provides an outline individual management plan wherever possible to ensure that the patient has an outline individual management plan, which gives the reason for treatment, agreed treatment programme and the planned duration. This plan should be consistent with any agreed shared-care protocols*

vi. *Keeps records – to maintain adequate records of the service provided, incorporating all known information relating to any significant events, e.g. adverse reactions, hospital admissions and relevant deaths of which the practice has been notified*

vii. *Ensures primary care staff training – each practice must ensure that all staff involved in providing any aspect of care under this scheme have the necessary training and skills to do so. Practices should be able to demonstrate that they have in place a policy to cover staff training and maintenance of skills*

viii. *Provides safe and suitable facilities for undertaking invasive procedures – LHBs should be satisfied that practices undertaking to provide the Gonadorelin Administration Enhanced Service have adequate and appropriate facilities and equipment comparable to those required for the safe provision of any invasive procedure."*

It is also worth mentioning here that we need to be clear what it is we are willing and able to provide and may want to provide before we get into discussions with the PCO. Too often, some of us go into these meetings with only a vague idea of what we want the service specification to look like. We are more likely to be unhappy with the final service specification if we leave this important part of our preparations until we enter the room.

Untoward events

This is an area that many new enhanced service specifications now contain. I suspect that because these are fairly new arrangements in many areas, this is a bit of risk management by the PCO to help identify major problems early. I don't think it causes us problems. You need to watch out, however, because some PCOs want you to tell them about any problems that may occur to the patients even if it has nothing to do with the enhanced service. Just make sure that reporting of adverse events is relevant to the service being provided. The model specification for administering gonadorelins included this paragraph:

"It is a condition of participation in this NES that practitioners will give notification, within 72 hours, of the information becoming known to him/her, to the LHB clinical governance lead, of all relevant significant adverse events, emergency admissions or deaths of any patient treated under this service. This is in addition to any statutory obligations."

Accreditation

Now this is an area you have to watch like a hawk! Many PCOs will try to put huge obstacles in your way – hoops to jump through, additional boxes to tick, certificates to get and courses to attend – so they can be sure you are able to do the job clinically. (The fact that it helps to cover their own backs may also have something to do with it.)

I am always fascinated by the fact that when we were doing these things for free, or under duress, no-one ever checked to see whether we were qualified to do it, or had been on the latest course or had a piece of paper to say that someone, somewhere felt we were safe to be involved. But as soon as we demand resources and as soon as they have to pay for something, they are under an 'obligation' to ensure standards.

You have to be very careful here not to agree to such onerous requirements to be allowed to provide a service that you end up scaring off everyone who might have been interested in the first place. You may wish to agree to an annual update course or a specific qualification or certificate; that is up to you and the service being commissioned.

You might also want to consider using appraisal as the baseline. This means that each doctor is professionally responsible for ensuring they have the skills, training, etc. to be able to provide the service carefully. This places the responsibility to keep up to date on the doctor but, then again, that is exactly where it should be. The model specification for administering gonadorelins included this paragraph:

"Doctors will need to satisfy, at appraisal, that they have the necessary medical experience, training and competence necessary to enable them to provide for a safe and effective gonadorelin enhanced service."

Pricing

This is perhaps the tricky one. The price accepted will depend on the costs of provision, any additional training, staff or equipment needs, and how much the other side has to play with. This is often why the prices for a seemingly similar service may vary from place to place. It does not mean that the best negotiators always get the best price because often you may accept a lower price to establish a much wanted precedent, or you may be looking to the next negotiation, or an even longer long game.

Direct comparisons are useful up to a point and you should do a search to see what kinds of fees others have agree to in other parts of the UK so you know your market place better. But the pricing section should at least include:

- The overall price of the contract
- How the payments are to be made, i.e. per patient, per block of patients, per year
- How the payments are made to your bank account
- Whether payments will be in advance or retrospective
- On what basis payments will be increased annually.

The model specification for administering gonadorelins included the following paragraphs:

"Given the different modes of administering gonadorelins for carcinoma of the prostate, an annual fee has been set for 2005/6 for providing an individual treatment package for patients as set out in the service outline of this specification.

The annual fees applicable are: all patients entering the scheme will attract an annual fee of £100, which will be payable quarterly in arrears, provided that at least one injection has been given in the relevant quarter. Existing patients, with an established diagnosis of carcinoma of the prostate, who require continuation of their gonadorelin treatment beyond 2005 will be regarded as new patients entering the scheme and will attract an annual retention fee of £100, which is payable quarterly in arrears, provided the patient has received at least one injection in the relevant quarter."

CHAPTER 7

HOW TO WORK OUT THE PRICE OF AN ENHANCED SERVICE

This is probably one of the areas that GPs are weakest at when it comes to negotiating an enhanced service. Many will look at the £100 payment in their hand and think they are £100 better off. This might be the case, especially if the staff and other costs of providing the service have been absorbed in GMS before the new contract. Many enhanced services may not need new staff or new equipment, and so the £100 is £100 of pure profit. But in many other cases we need to incur new costs to provide the services. This can be extra staff time, training costs, premises costs, etc. We need to make sure that we don't spend £105 earning £100 and think we've done well!

When setting the price for a service, whatever the nature, there are several factors you need to take into account. I have given some examples in **Box 3**. When most people start this type of local negotiation, they simply pick a number in their mind and then aim for that. They often do not think of the underlying costs to the practice of providing the service, seeing only the cash coming in, ignoring the expenses going out. If you do this you may end up losing money, not gaining it.

BOX 3	FACTORS TO CONSIDER WHEN PRICING A SERVICE

- The cost to you of providing the service
- Any alternative providers in the locality
- How much you 'want' to provide the service
- How much the PCO 'wants' you to provide the service
- Alternative services you may want to or be asked to provide
- The inconvenience factor in providing the service
- Market value of the service, i.e. how much other people are providing the service for, both locally and nationally
- Hidden costs to you of providing the service
- Hidden costs to the PCO of alternative providers, e.g. ambulance transport if provided by the PCO or trust

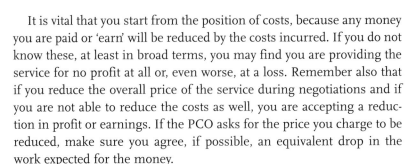

It is vital that you start from the position of costs, because any money you are paid or 'earn' will be reduced by the costs incurred. If you do not know these, at least in broad terms, you may find you are providing the service for no profit at all or, even worse, at a loss. Remember also that if you reduce the overall price of the service during negotiations and if you are not able to reduce the costs as well, you are accepting a reduction in profit or earnings. If the PCO asks for the price you charge to be reduced, make sure you agree, if possible, an equivalent drop in the work expected for the money.

A simple pro forma for working out the costs expected and the profit wanted is given in Appendix 6 and Appendix 7, respectively. I have discussed the main areas to look at below.

How to calculate the costs element of a contract

Practice staff

When estimating practice staff costs don't forget the additional costs of employing staff, e.g. national insurance, pension contributions, training costs, holidays, sickness, maternity leave and other 'replacement' costs.

New staff

Do you need to take on new staff, such as a healthcare assistant or receptionist? Are there skills you need or that you will need to bring in? This is not always about employing new highly trained or skilled people. We can often delegate existing work to new staff or employ staff to take on work that requires lower technical skills. For example, healthcare assistants can do routine blood pressure monitoring or ECGs, freeing up more skilled staff (such as nurses).

Extending staff hours

Can existing staff work more hours? This may save you the time and cost of advertising, recruiting, training, etc.

Training staff

You may need to train staff for particular aspects of the service. As well as the cost of the training, you may need to consider the cost of backfill or replacing the staff when they are away being trained. If you don't build these in, you will be paying for them out of your own profit.

Additional medico-legal cover

Many practices now include their practice staff in their medical defence cover. These practice policies may need to be updated or reviewed if staff start to provide a higher level of skilled work, or if new staff join the practice. If a new service requires new skills or staff it is important to find out from your medical defence organisation whether there will be additional costs. These must then make up part of the expense element of your agreed price.

Equipment

New equipment
An example of a service that is likely to need new equipment is INR monitoring, where the test itself is done at the practice. You must build this into the service cost. And don't forget any ongoing costs outlined below. If you don't factor them in, you may find that your first year or so of profit is simply buying you a machine to do the work.

Training for using equipment
As well as the cost of training, time taken to learn how to use equipment has a cost either in direct time or backfill, replacement costs.

Running costs
You need to factor in the running and maintenance costs for the whole year. For example an ECG uses paper, a test machine will often need cleaner and calibration fluids, etc.

I know this sounds a bit petty, but for every cost you don't consider and get funding for, the less you will be earning. You need only a few of these 'little' costs to make a sizeable dent in your annual profit for the enhanced service. There is nothing quite so discouraging than to work all year only to find you've earned a pittance, even before tax, national insurance and pension contributions.

Insurance and contract costs
Insurance costs would include things like contents cover.

Premises

Do you need to build, extend or improve your premises? If so, you could build in some of the expense into the cost of provision. The question to ask is, could you provide the service safely if you don't improve your premises?

As well as direct costs, you need to consider running costs, such as electricity and heating, decoration costs, and the cost of consumables.

Doctors

If a GP is doing the work for the enhanced service, they cannot be doing other work, e.g. providing essential work. If they are doing the work in 'non-essential' time then it has to be paid for. If they are doing the work during 'essential services' time then there is usually a backfill cost that the practice will incur to replace the provider doctor. These costs have to be factored in. Replacing doctors is not cheap!

As with practice staff, there may be additional or ongoing training costs and corresponding locum backfill costs.

Additional medico-legal cover

Don't assume that the work is covered by your existing medical defence policy; it's better to check now than find out later that your defence organisation refuses to cover you later. Even if there are no additional costs there is nothing wrong in getting the commissioner to pay for a proportion of your defence costs because you would not be able to provide the service without it.

How to calculate the profit element of a contract

There are several ways of working out what you would like to earn from providing a service. There is no 'right way' as such, and there are various approaches you can take. You need to choose the method most suited to you and the service. The main point here is not how you arrive at the number, but that the number is adequate and represents a decent income for proving the service.

It is worth mentioning that because we are now responsible for the full pension contributions on NHS work we need to make sure that any fee we agree takes this into account. In the past, as 'employees' we contributed 6% of our income to our pensions and the 'employer' (the PCO for this purpose) contributed a further 14% – a total of 20%. Because we are now responsible for the full 20% on any NHS profits we make we must make sure that this additional 14% that we need to contribute is accounted for in the fees and payments for any enhanced service we provide.

Option 1: use a standard percentage of the total contract price

Under the old Red Book arrangements, we used to work out income and expenses and generally used an expense to earnings ratio of roughly 60:40, although this varied between practices. Basically, this meant that when we were paid £100, £60 of that was spent by us to provide the service leaving £40 as profit or earnings. This level varied between practices for all sorts of reasons, but generally this was the ballpark figure.

Using this method of calculating potential profit, profits are set at 66% of costs. In other words, if the cost to you to provide the service is £100 then the figure you should ask for is £166. Once you have estimated the costs to you of providing the service, you could use this sort of calculation to arrive at a final figure or overall cost to the commissioner for you to provide the service required.

Option 2: use identifiable doctor hours

Some enhanced services may have little in the way of additional or identifiable costs to the practice. This would include areas where the practice has been offering the service for a while, and the expenses have been absorbed into the global sum (or minimum practice income guarantee) because they were there before the new contract. In this case you may decide to simply value the profit you want to achieve based on the number of hours the doctors and other staff work to provide the service.

It is worth remembering that in this case, any additional funding coming in would be almost 100% profit. But as I have mentioned above, don't forget the employers' superannuation contributions that we are now responsible for getting from the PCO (as part of the fees paid) and making to the pensions agency.

Option 3: decide a set amount of profit to be earned

Some GPs may just want to earn a certain amount for proving the service. In this case you should simply set the amount you want to earn after identifiable costs. This may reflect workload, intensity, your interest in the disease or service area, etc. (These are not the only three factors, but they are the most common I have used or come across.)

A summary of these potential methods is given in Appendix 7.

Superannuation

As I have mentioned earlier, you must remember that any profit that can be classified as NHS work is now superannuable under the NHS scheme. With the commencement of the new contract all NHS work can be superannuated. But GPs are now responsible for the 6% employee's contribution that we have always had to pay and the 14% that used to be termed employer's contributions.

Some of this employer's superannuation has been included in the global sum uplift added in April 2004 and to the quality and outcome framework pounds per point from the same date. But even then there is a known shortfall between the amount the GPC felt needed to be added and the actual amount added by the government. You need to make sure that the additional 14% for which we are now responsible is contained within the price. If you don't you will in effect be giving yourself a pay cut.

Work that qualifies under the new contract as pensionable is given in **Box 4.**

BOX 4	**PENSIONABLE WORK UNDER THE NEW CONTRACT**

- The net profits derived from the payments made to GPs in respect of NHS work, i.e. the delivery of direct patient care under GMS or personal medical services arrangements
- Board advisory work or other work carried out for PCOs or other health services bodies
- Work carried out for social services under the collaborative arrangements
- Work carried out while educating or organising the education of medical students and undergraduates and postgraduate training funded through national levies or otherwise
- Work under the requirements of Schedule 9 of the NHS (General Medical Services) Regulations 1992 as amended and their four other country equivalents
- Locum work
- Any other NHS work

CHAPTER 8
HOW TO SAY 'NO' TO UNWANTED OR UNRESOURCED WORK

This chapter first appeared as an article in *Doctor* magazine right at the start of the contract implementation process. I use it with their kind permission. It may seem a little dated now but I think the principles are still valid.

How to say 'no' ... and mean it

One of the strongest messages from GPs before the new contract negotiations was that we felt we had lost of control of our workload. So one of the main changes needed in the new contract was the ability for GPs to say 'no' to new work and to opt out of workload we felt unable to provide.

We have always had the right to say 'no' to workload shift, but many of us have been afraid to do so. We have been afraid of threats made by health authorities and PCOs, of being seen as a 'bad' doctor or person if we said 'no' or that our patients might not receive the care they need unless we took on the work. Our highly developed sense of responsibility towards our patients has given others, with less sense of that responsibility, the opportunity to dump work onto GPs, without any thought of resourcing us.

Here, I have suggested how GPs can say 'no' to new work and how to prepare to opt out of workload before and after 1 April 2004. I need to make it clear that these are my personal thoughts and feelings and in no way represent BMA policy or advice.

After saying 'yes', admittedly reluctantly, to new work for such a long time, and suddenly realising that we are now able to say 'no', the risk is that we will do so in an unplanned and chaotic manner that will not be good for our patients or us. That is not to say we keep saying 'yes', far from it, but it is my experience that planned withdrawal from this work, or planned negotiation of payment works best.

There are three areas to consider:
- The inevitable attempts by others to shift work our way with no thought of a properly commissioned service, which includes funding arrangements

- The workload we have already taken on and from which we may wish to withdraw before 1 April 2004
- The workload we want to withdraw from after April 2004.

I'll deal with each one of these in turn.

How to say 'no' to workload creep

First, practise saying 'no'. It isn't as easy as it sounds and many of us, by our own admission, are not comfortable doing so. It is worth starting with something easy that won't directly affect patient care. For example, my practice recently received a letter from a trust asking us to agree that after a patient had received ionising radiation in its area, we would accept responsibility to inform the district nurse team leader so she could inform her staff (all employed by the same trust). We wrote back stating that because the trust retained the employer responsibility to inform its staff of any risks to their health and that the more steps in the communication chain, the more likely it was to break down, we could not and should not accept the responsibility. We formally refused. We have heard nothing since.

This is a simple example but similar to ones commonly described by GPs up and down the country. There are usually several very good reasons why we can say 'no'.

1. We may not have the clinical skills to provide the service

A patient once asked me to take off their ingrown toenail. I have never done one so said I wouldn't be able to. The patient, bless their heart, understood this but asked if I could 'have a go'! I suggested that my 'having a go' would neither be in their or my best interests! Many things we are asked to do, we are not trained to do. This doesn't mean we can refuse to keep up to date, or refuse all progress in patient care, but there are treatments that GPs are simply not trained to a sufficient level to do. I have never prescribed methadone, even under extreme pressure from different parties, because I don't feel I have the skills to undertake this treatment.

It is more difficult for others to try to force us to take on work when we have made it very clear that we don't feel clinically able to take over or provide the treatment. Give the other side a formal notification as outlined above and ask them to formally state that they understand your concerns. This often helps them reconsider whether they are ready to accept the responsibility of sending patients to someone who has clearly said they don't have the needed skills. The General Medical Council might be interested in this.

2. We should ask for the resources for the work to be transferred to us now

The work is already being done somewhere and someone is being paid to do it. If the work moves then the money should follow. This request alone unsettles the other side, but only if they are sure that you won't do the work for free. The fact that they have to identify the money and move it will often stop, or at least delay, the workload shift until the appropriate arrangements can be made. If they send the work anyway, my habit is to write immediately to the patient and the 'sender' explaining that, as discussed before, I am unable to provide this work. It is a bit of a nuisance, but you need only do this once or twice. It is much better if you can coordinate together a large group of practices, for example via the LMC.

3. The effect on your current patients would be detrimental

We should resist anything that may affect our ability to provide the top-quality service we want to provide for our patients. Even our initial refusal forces the other side to find reasons (other than 'well, you have to do it, you're the GP') why you should take the work on. It is quite amusing to read some of the arguments put forward. These are usually very weak and can be argued against very easily, strengthening your position.

4. We are often not the most appropriate person to do the work

There are often other people in the NHS who can do certain work better or more efficiently than us. The other side won't have approached these people because it would mean commissioning (and funding) the service from, say, a trust or hospital, which have considerable expertise at saying 'no' unless money follows. If they come to you because they think they'll get the service for free, saying 'no' and explaining why will often make them think again.

Getting into the habit of saying 'no' often, and backing this up with good, reasoned arguments strengthens our position and forces the other party to defend theirs.

How to opt out of work you have previously taken on without payment or resourcing

First, decide whether you really want to opt out completely or whether you want to provide the service if you are paid for it. It is good for the other side to know whether they are supposed to be negotiating over payment or discussing when you are going to opt out of the work.

In the mid 1990s the General Medical Services Committee proposed the GMS core/non-core strategy. This paper, accepted by the LMC conference, was the first attempt by GPs to limit their workload by defining what was part of GMS and what was not. It listed many services not considered to be GMS. It was this paper that encouraged many of us to start developing LDSs. Some areas have been very successful at setting up LDSs, whereas others have been less so. There are many reasons why this occurred including whether the health authority saw the potential of LDSs in developing patient services, whether the local GPs were united in their work and whether they were 'aggressive' in their negotiations, for example including the option of opting out without a set agreement.

Many PCOs have used all sorts of threats against GPs to prevent them from asking for fair funding for services provided. These threats become less important when you are part of a large group of GPs. If threatened, I ask for it to be put in writing so 'I can check the legal background to their position'. This rarely comes. So I record exactly what was said by whom, where and in what context, because you never know when you might need it.

Remember, many GPs are being paid for these services now. This is an acceptance by the NHS that these services are *not* GMS. This has to be the case or the NHS would be paying us for the same work twice, once via GMS and again via the LDS. This would be illegal. So the fact that these services are being paid for throughout the country, means that the NHS has tacitly agreed we are not currently contracted to provide them. If we are not contracted to provide them, I believe we can stop providing them as long as we transfer their care to someone with the necessary skills, e.g. the local medical or haematology department.

Box 5 lists some LDSs that are currently being paid for (although it is not an exhaustive list). The GPC is compiling a nationwide list of LDSs currently in place. This will be available to all LMCs and GPs.

So how do we go about this?

BOX 5	LOCAL DEVELOPMENT SCHEMES ACTIVE IN THE UK

- Warfarin monitoring
- Named shared-care drug monitoring
- Lithium monitoring
- Nursing homes (additional services to GMS)
- Asylum seekers (additional services to GMS)
- Services to violent patients
- Drug misuse substitution prescribing

Step 1

First decide what you want to stop or get paid for providing. This distinction is important for you and the other side when starting discussions. Practices can do this individually, as a group or across an LMC area.

Step 2

I would then suggest immediately discussing with your local practices and/or the LMC how others feel and, if possible, working together. It is worth the LMC writing to all practices to ask whether they would like the LMC to negotiate on their behalf and getting the remit for negotiations. It is more difficult for the PCO to refuse to discuss something that all GPs want them to deal with.

Step 3

Next, find examples of other GPs getting paid for this work. This stops the other side saying that no-one else gets paid and gives you the details of current schemes, requirements and pay scales that have already been negotiated.

Step 4

Inform the PCO either that you want to stop providing the service or to agree an LDS for the work. I feel three months' notice of your intent to cease providing the service, or for reaching an agreement, is reasonable.

The PCO will do one of two things:

- Agree to meet and discuss your request, in which case you have a negotiation
- Refuse to meet (or try to delay a meeting) in an attempt to avoid a discussion. They know they don't have the moral high ground here, so it is difficult for most managers (but not all) to try to argue why you should work very hard for free.

Step 5

If they refuse to meet, you need to move up a gear. There are several ways this has been done in the past.

- Write to the local patients' organisation. Outline the problems you are facing and the resources you need. Send copies of the letters you have sent to the PCO and the negative responses you have received. Think carefully about this one; your decision whether to do this may depend on how supportive your local group has been in the past.
- Write to the local hospital trust explaining that because of lack of progress with the PCO it is likely that the work will be referred back

to them in a few months. Suggest that they start discussions soon with the PCO about their requirements for funding.

- Use the small claims court. If you inform someone that there is a charge for the work, and they still send the work to you, you are entitled to send them a bill. The PCO will probably refuse to pay it, so you can then take them to small claims court. Keep the bill under the limit for the small claims court (currently under £3000). You need to inform the PCO of your intentions should it not reach an agreement, refuse to pay you or not tell you where to refer patients for the services it needs. I did this right at the start of the LDS process and found it very useful. If the PCO refuses to pay but attends the court hearing, it will have to prove that the work is part of current GMS – an impossible task as described earlier. I have never had to actually go to the small claims court, but was really looking forward to seeing the chief executive of the health authority trying to justify the authority's position.

- Write to your patients explaining that the service may be transferred if the PCO is unable to fund the service from the practice in the future. Patients understand that we are very busy and under pressure, and they are often very helpful at supporting the aims of the practice. Patient petitions and letters can be useful but, again, think how to best use this avenue. It is worth reminding patients that if the service is provided by the hospital in the future, they may qualify for ambulance transport.

- Informing the ambulance trust of this potential future demand will help their forward planning.

There are other people and organisations you may want to consider involving, depending on local circumstances. The key is not to feel defensive when refusing work. It is not yours to start with. The key is to make the other side defend and explain its positions giving reasons why it feels it shouldn't pay you for the work.

The usual reason given is that the PCO has no money. What a load of old nonsense! The NHS is always paying for services it 'can't afford'. But it seems that it's OK to overspend on services provided by hospitals, even by many millions of pounds, but it's very much not OK to overspend on general practice. Imagine what could be provided if even a small portion of the secondary care overspend was spent in general practice. Areas where these schemes have been set up often find there is no money until it becomes clear that the GPs will stop services. Funnily enough, the money is usually then found.

I believe that all GPs can follow this process, because some of us have been doing just that for the past six or seven years. However, remember that if you have a current contract for providing enhanced services (or LDSs) you must complete or renegotiate that contract.

How to opt out of services after April 2004

This is much easier. The new contract makes it very clear that we are contracted to provide essential services and the additional services we agreed to provide at the start of the contractual process. This may vary between practices. It also makes it clear that anything that does not fall into these two categories is not part of our contract and so we have no obligation to provide it. The list of NESs was given in Box 2 (see page 4).

We don't have to fight a big battle here; that has already been done. If the PCO is not willing to enter into negotiations or offer a contract for enhanced services, we are under no obligation to provide them. You simply say that because it has not offered you a new contract for these services, in line with the new contract, you will cease to provide the service from 1 April 2004. (Remember the three-month notice period I discussed earlier. So if you decide to opt out on 1 April 2004, you should give notice at least by 1 January 2004.) The PCO is then obliged to provide the service or commission the service from other providers. And if it will pay someone else to provide the service, questions need to be asked!

Summary

During the new contract negotiations, the ability to control workload was at or near the top of most GPs' wish lists. Now that we can opt out of work, we must be prepared to do it. Saying 'no, ... well, OK then' will help no-one. Don't feel defensive about saying 'no'. There are good reasons why we cannot take on the work or why we cannot take it on without adequate resources.

Make the other side defend its position when asking us to work harder and harder for nothing. Look for natural allies. Be prepared to be the bad guys in some people's eyes; the hassle is worth it in the long run. Other sections of the NHS have been saying 'we don't do that' for years. In many cases it shows that you are the most responsible person involved. Seek help early on, from other practices in your area, the LMC or the GPC. I am always happy to advise when asked, so please feel free.

The new contract can help protect us against slavery, but nothing can protect us against ourselves if we give in and agree to voluntary slavery.

CHAPTER 9
BASIC NEGOTIATING SKILLS

In this chapter, if you will excuse the self-indulgence, I have borrowed from my book *Successful Negotiation in the New Contract* (Butterworth Heinemann, 2004). I have included seven 'crib sheets' from the relevant chapters of that book for reference. Each crib sheet covers a different aspect of negotiating. I have also added a section on 'principled negotiating' to offer an alternative style of negotiating.

I wrote the book on negotiating skills because many GPs say they don't have them, and feel intimidated when faced with a potential negotiation such as for developing enhanced services. The truth, though, is that almost all of us have some basic skills but we don't always recognise them as such.

Anyone can do it

The first thing to realise is that negotiation is something we all do every day. A negotiation can be described simply as where two people or two sides start from different places, with different wants and wishes, and end up agreeing on a way forward that is acceptable to both sides. All of us have basic negotiating skills. There is nothing special about negotiating. It is a series of skills and techniques that, like most things in life, come more naturally to some of us than others. But these skills and techniques can be learned and developed by all of us. All it takes is some training and practice. To be honest, we all begin to learn these basic skills of negotiating as children.

For example, those of you with teenaged children will quickly recognise the negotiating you often need to do with them to either get them to do the things you want or to stop the behaviour you don't want. In these often simple (?!) negotiations we use many different techniques, for example we will often prepare what we are going to say, and how we are going to say it; we anticipate their concerns, moans and whinges. We then use persuasion, evidence, expertise, moral high ground, threats and many other negotiating techniques and ploys to try to bring them around to our way of thinking. Be careful though, because we all know they will often try to do the exact same thing to us in an attempt to bring us around to their way of thinking! Hopefully we agree a way forward and both sides then follow up to make sure the other side does what it agreed to do. If any side fails in their obligations, the negotiations usually start all over again. I can't say that reading this book will make you a better parent, but who knows.

Again, most of us who work as principal GPs will have some experience at trying to negotiate discounts with drug companies on the vaccines and other drugs we use in our surgeries. Once again, we use the basic skills of negotiation, often without noticing that that is exactly what we are doing. We prepare by finding out the discounts that others may have been able to get from the company, or what other companies may be ready to offer us. We explore not just the price but the additional benefits, such as the return policies of the company on unused stock. We will often look at a deal covering more than one year and look to improve the deal over the longer term by offering them want they want, which is a deal and agreement over several years. And we do all this before we sign on the dotted line. So we use the basic skills of negotiation every day even if we don't always see or recognise them as such.

I don't want to labour the point too much, but I'd like to emphasise that everyone has some degree of skill in this area. The thing to remember is that negotiating is something we do all the time. All of us can develop and improve the basic skills we have by recognising what we are doing right and what we are doing wrong and then practising.

The following sections follow the usual step-by-step process most negotiating teams I have been a member of use to try to ensure the best deal they can get in any situation. These steps are:

- Preparation
- The meeting itself
- Finishing the negotiation
- Follow up.

I will outline each step in some detail, including how to prepare for the negotiation by gathering evidence, doing research and trying to predict the opposite party's worries and concerns. Then, by developing your combined individual and team skills of negotiation, it will be easier to know when you have got as far as you are going to get this time, know when to close the negotiation and establish appropriate follow up to ensure both sides do what they said they would do.

If you follow the process and the steps outlined you will have a much better grasp of the basics and therefore a far better chance of reaching a good outcome from each separate negotiation. It's just like how we learn in medical school. We are taught examination as a series of steps. We are constantly reminded that if you follow each step in turn each time you examine someone, you will be much less likely to miss anything important and far more likely to pick up the signs and symptoms of disease. Negotiation is also a series of steps and behaviours, which can be learnt and, if followed, can improve our chances of not missing out on anything important or valuable.

Negotiation is a specific activity with a specific purpose. It is meant to bring two sides to a mutually agreed position by each side giving something in exchange for something else they want. Negotiation is often confused with other things, for example:

- Consultation
- Arbitration
- Discussions or exchanging views
- Exploring options.

These have different roles and functions. The end result is different. Before you enter into a negotiation, make sure both sides realise what it is you are doing and that the expectations of both sides match! The following seven crib sheets will guide you through different aspects of negotiating.

1 CRIB SHEET

What to do before you get in the room

- Be clear what you want to provide and what you do not want to provide.
- Decide what you are prepared to concede or give away, and in what order of priority.
- Honestly assess your strengths. If you cannot think of any, ask around.
- Assess your weaknesses. Think laterally, as the other side would, to identify your potential weaker areas. Prepare your defences for each one.
- Work out all the financial and other costs that would be incurred if you provide the service.
- Use all financial expertise to do this (e.g. practice manager and accountant).
- Decide what level of profit you want to earn from providing the service. Again, use your financial advisers to help you with this.
- Spend time working out what the other side is likely to want. Use initial contacts with them to try to work this out.
- Identify alternative providers the other side could use.
- Identify any external pressures the other side may be under to reach an agreement with you.
- Find out who is on their team and what you know about them.
- Remember that you are not powerless. Power is about what your options are, what you can do to exert pressure on the other side and what they feel you might do if they do not reach a settlement with you. The perception of power can be as useful as real power itself.
- If the problem is fear, then the cure is preparation.

2	CRIB SHEET

Prepare for the meeting itself

- Make sure that all the members of your team know what the team's aims are.
- Decide roles before meeting with the other side. These roles can vary between different meetings and even within a meeting. One person can have more than one role, but should not have more than two.
- The roles you need to assign are:
  - Speaker
  - Recorder
  - Compass
  - Watcher/listener.
- Make sure you know how long the meeting is planned to last. If you feel you need longer, don't be afraid to say so before the meeting.
- Each meeting should have an aim in terms of outcomes. If you know what you want, you're more likely to get it.
- Agree the agenda before the meeting.
- Don't leave important items to the end of the agenda.
- If the other side wants to change the agenda once the meeting has started, make sure you agree to the changes and the (real) reasons for the change.
- In the meeting, listen to what is said and not said.
- 'Hear' the messages.

3 CRIB SHEET

The meeting itself: basic skills

- Try to get the other side to open the meeting with their position.
- Listen to what they say without giving an immediate response.
- Use questions to elicit further information from them. The more you know before you make your response the better.
- When you respond, do so calmly.
- If you open first, do so confidently. You are the experts at what you do, so be confident.
- Don't show all your cards at this stage, keep a few up your sleeve for later.
- Be firm, aim high and be credible.
- Use as many negotiating skills and techniques as you feel confident with.
- Don't use the same negotiating technique all the time.
- Remember, practice makes perfect. Don't be afraid to experiment.

4   CRIB SHEET

Things to avoid, or not touch with a barge pole!

- Don't blurt anything out, even if it seems a good idea. Let your speaker know of your idea or thought, and between you decide whether it would warrant a time out.
- If you disagree with something your speaker or another team member has said, don't argue in front of the other side; let your colleague know via a note.
- Don't take things personally.
- Don't argue or try to score cheap points.
- Compromise late in the process and do it slowly.
- Don't give ranges for the other side to choose from. They will always choose the lowest or least beneficial to you. Always give specifics.
- Beware of the 'meet in the middle' ploy. This tends to favour the side that takes the most extreme position early on. Don't be swayed by the 'well it would be fair to both sides' argument.
- If you get a good win or a gain, don't show triumph. It will set the other side against more gains in the future.
- Always say 'thank you' for each gain. It will help you to stop showing triumph and is good manners.
- Don't let the other side take you down paths you don't want to go down.
- Follow the discussions at all times. If the other side sees you drift, they might try to slip something small but important past you.
- If something seems too good to be true, it usually is.
- Attempts to overtly intimidate usually fail, but if you do succeed then you will put their backs up and you may pay later on. No-one likes to feel threatened, so if you have to, do it gently.
- Remember, it's easy to get everything you want if you want nothing. If you end the negotiation with everything you set out to get, then you may just have aimed too low. Re-evaluate for the next time.

5   CRIB SHEET

At the end – don't lose any gains you have made by sloppiness now

- It may be time to stop the negotiation to see whether it is worth taking what is on offer when:
  - You seem to have a lot of what you want
  - The distance between you and the other side is growing increasingly small
  - The arguments get fewer and fewer and over smaller and smaller things.
- Make sure you summarise at the end to ensure each side is clear about what has been agreed.
- Record everything.
- Write the summary down and let both sides have the same record.
- If you have a piece of work to do before the next meeting, do it well.
- Do all assigned work on time if possible. This will increase your own confidence and theirs in you.
- Build on success, take the time to appreciate where you are and plan the next steps you want to take.
- There will be many negotiations; you will do better on some than others. Don't worry, this is just how it is.
- Remember that we learn more from mistakes than success, especially about who our friends are.

6 CRIB SHEET

How to say 'no'

- The inability to control our workload was one of the most common complaints of the old Red Book.
- Negotiation is not just about getting paid; it is about getting paid well, or walking away.
- GPs are often concerned about saying 'no' for various reasons. We have the same rights to work or not work as the rest of the population.
- We are not responsible for all the NHS services that our patients need, just that bit we are contracted for.
- If you decide to walk away or stop providing a service, it is best to do it in an orderly and structured way. This will keep others on your side as much as possible.
- Make sure the other side is in no doubt that you have an exit strategy that includes not agreeing a deal and withdrawing from providing the services, if you are already doing so.
- Bluffs can work, but you look pretty silly if they call, and you fold.
- Inform those organisations that may be affected by your decision to withdraw, in enough time to allow them to make changes if needed.
- Keep the LMC involved and informed at all stages.
- Don't feel defensive about saying 'no'. You have the same rights as everyone else in the NHS to earn a living and have a life at the same time. Don't let anyone tell you otherwise. You are only selling them your time and skills, not your soul!

7 CRIB SHEET

Learn from each negotiation

- Learning is a life-long pursuit. Don't expect to get it right each and every time.
- Resist the temptation to apportion blame to one or two people. Negotiating is a team effort and should be a team learning exercise.
- Review all aspects of your preparation. Remember good sources of ideas and information for future negotiations.
- Review what worked and what did not.
- Look at team roles. Did you keep to them? Were you better suited for other roles?
- Look at team discipline. Were you disciplined?
- Examine the meeting itself. Was it as you planned or did it go off in strange directions?
- Did you get to present all your work or did the other side limit your time? If the latter, read about negotiating techniques for getting back on track.
- Did the agenda do its job? Did you use it to its maximum benefits?
- Did you have fun?

Principled negotiating

Many organisations' negotiating teams have been trained in negotiating skills according to the principled negotiating model as expounded in Fisher and Ury's book *Getting to Yes: Negotiating an Agreement Without Giving In* (Arrow, 1997). Those who don't follow this model are often offended by the title 'principled negotiating' because it might imply that someone who does not follow the model is unprincipled or is following an unprincipled negotiating method. For those who feel this way, an alternative name is 'negotiating on the merits'.

I wanted to include this section, based on a paper put together by Justin Cross of the GPC, to give an initial and alternative view of negotiating and an insight into the model of principled negotiating in order to understand its approach and protocols for negotiation.

What principled negotiating is not

Principled negotiating is not positional bargaining. Positional bargaining can be defined as the successive taking and then giving up of a sequence of positions. Fisher and Ury suggest that there are three criteria for fairly judging a negotiating method. It should:

- Produce a wise agreement if agreement is possible (a wise agreement is one that meets the legitimate interests of each side to the greatest extent possible, resolves conflicting interests, is durable and takes community interests into account)
- Be efficient
- Improve, or at least not damage, the relationship between the parties.

Some people worry about positional negotiating because they feel it does not always produce the best results. Some of their concerns are that positional bargaining:

- Does not always produce wise agreements because the parties haggle over positions, which they attack and defend. These positions can become entrenched: the more one side tries to convince the other to change, the more impossible it becomes for you to change
- Can be seen as inefficient. It wastes time because it may provide incentives that hinder reaching an agreement
- May endanger ongoing relationships because it often becomes a battle of wills in which someone has to give in and someone has to win.

Furthermore, positional bargaining can be more difficult when engaging in multiparty negotiations or where the negotiators represent constituencies because it is more difficult to find common positions, and once positions have been agreed it is more difficult to amend them subsequently.

There are two ways of playing positional bargaining: the hard way and the soft way. The *hard way* involves negotiating against adversaries with the intention of winning, demanding concessions, being distrustful, making threats, intentionally misleading and digging in on one's position. It rarely produces a wise agreement that is *acceptable to both or all parties.*

The *soft way* involves negotiating with friends to reach agreement, making concessions, avoiding conflict and confrontation, changing position easily and yielding to pressure. It rarely produces a wise agreement that is *acceptable to both or all parties.*

What is principled negotiating?

Principled negotiating is not positional bargaining and it is not negotiating the hard way or the soft way. Principled negotiating can be simplified into four key points as shown in **Box 6**.

BOX 6	PRINCIPLED NEGOTIATING: FOUR KEY POINTS

- Separate the people from the problem
- Focus on interests, not positions
- Invent options for mutual gain
- Insist on using objective criteria

The problem not the people

People have emotions and egos that become attached to the positions they espouse in negotiations. By focusing on the issue rather than the people, discussions are less emotionally charged and there is less political capital to forgo if one is asking the other party to change their mind about the issue. The process of negotiation should be joint problem solving.

Interests not positions

The outcome of a negotiation should satisfy the parties' underlying interests. It is essential to explore these interests, principally by asking questions, because this way is more likely to identify the common ground between the parties, which is likely to be greater than originally expected. Negotiating positions often obscure these interests and the common ground. By seeking to reach an agreement that deals with these interests you solve the underlying problem rather than merely treating the symptom as expressed by the negotiating positions.

Be creative

If the parties are working together to satisfy their interests, they can be creative about the solution that will maximise the outcome for both or all parties. Rather than choosing an option from a predetermined list of possible solutions developed by one party or the other, better solutions can be explored and found, outside what may have been the original or obvious answers, which satisfy everyone.

Use objective criteria

A wise agreement is not one where one party concedes or where one party wins. A wise agreement must be seen to be such according to a fair independent standard and should not just reflect the position of one side. If both sides use objective criteria, this avoids creating winners and losers in the negotiating arena, which is essential if you are seeking a wise solution.

Conclusion

Both sides will have political capital wrapped up in the process and outcome. Therefore, it is essential to the success of the negotiation that neither side is put in a position of conceding. This is much easier to achieve if both parties are focusing on problem solving, attempting to satisfy underlying interests, being creative about the solution and able to defend the outcome objectively. There is a great deal of methodology to support this theory in practice. Suffice to say much of the focus is on preparation.

Introducing BATNAs

A BATNA, as described by Fisher and Ury, is a Best Alternative To a Negotiated Agreement.

What is a BATNA not?

It is not a bottom line. A bottom line appears to be a useful protection because it makes it easier to resist pressure and temptations of the moment. However, it limits your ability to benefit from what you have learnt during the negotiation, it inhibits imagination and is often set too high (Fisher and Ury). It is not conducive towards achieving a wise agreement.

It is not just determining when to walk away. Part of the BATNA is to know when not to reach agreement, but more importantly it is to know why.

What is a BATNA?

The purpose of entering negotiation is to achieve something more than could have been achieved without negotiation. To determine this, it is necessary to know what could be achieved without negotiation, i.e. the alternative(s). Only when you know the potential alternative results from not negotiating can you judge the acceptability of the outcome of a negotiation. The BATNA (the best alternative) is therefore the standard against which you measure a proposed agreement reached through negotiation.

The reason why this is better than a bottom line is because it stops you from rejecting terms that might satisfy your interests because it is sufficiently flexible to allow for imaginative solutions, while still protecting you from accepting something that is unfavourable (Fisher and Ury). Therefore, Fisher and Ury state:

- It is important to have determined what you will do in the event of no agreement
- Don't assume you have many alternatives. The costs of alternatives may be much higher
- Don't see all the alternatives in aggregate in comparison to a proposed agreement. You are likely to follow only one
- Don't be too committed to reach an agreement, explore alternatives
- Develop a trip wire. The trip wire is like a bottom line but is set at a level that would deliver a far from perfect agreement, but is better than your BATNA. This allows time for reflection and taking stock before getting too close to your BATNA
- Spend time formulating alternatives. As with wise agreements themselves, a BATNA is unlikely to be obvious and will need developmental work to be creative and explore options. The BATNA is the best of these options
- The better the BATNA, the greater the negotiating power because you will be comfortable knowing what the best alternative is (assuming there is an alternative)
- Consider the other negotiating party's BATNA(s). This will help you determine how strong your negotiating position is in comparison.

Preparing for negotiations

Consider the following points as part of your preparation for negotiation.

- Determine your negotiating objectives.
- Define your BATNA.
- Consider the other negotiating party's objectives and BATNA.
- For each of the issues to be covered in the negotiation, determine the minimum limit you would settle for, the target limit you are aiming for and what would be a satisfactory limit within that range. Furthermore, prioritise the issues.
- Determine what is not negotiable.
- Determine what the common ground is between the negotiating parties.
- Determine the questions you need to ask to gather necessary information and to explore interests.
- Determine which arguments to use (see section on 'reds and blues' later in the next section).
- Determine what information not to reveal, or when to reveal information.
- Explore and plan different scenarios to determine whether some are acceptable as a package.
- Decide which roles members of the negotiating team should play in the negotiation: the chairman, lead negotiator, person to lead the questions/explore the other side's interests, summariser, etc.

Reds and blues

Playing a 'red' or playing a 'blue' is shorthand. The terms are derived from a negotiating skills game, in which participants learn the value of trusting their negotiating partners and communicating that trust if they are to achieve a wise agreement to the mutual benefit of both parties.

In this context a red denotes putting forward an argument or offer that is honest and transparent, and that could be seen to be making yourself vulnerable. It is essentially asking the other negotiating party to trust you and to engage with you honestly and transparently. Their response should be also to play a red. In this circumstance, consecutive reds will become a virtuous circle leading to a creative, wise agreement satisfying the mutual interests of the parties.

Playing a blue denotes that you are proceeding cautiously and that on balance you do not trust the other negotiating party. It normally engenders an equally cautious and mistrustful response. So consecutive blues will become a vicious circle that leads to entrenched positions. It will be appropriate at times to play a blue as a defensive measure; for example if no positive responses ensue from the other side when you have played some consecutive reds.

CHAPTER 10
EXAMPLES OF ESTABLISHED ENHANCED SERVICES

I have included, in Appendix 8, a long list of established enhanced services cited in the library held by GPC UK. The list was correct at the time of writing, although I suspect others will have been added by now. I have also included some of these in full detail in Appendices 9–19. There are several reasons for including them.

First, we sometimes get the feeling that enhanced services are a waste of time and effort. Being able to see that in some areas very good enhanced services have been established helps us to realise what can be and has been achieved. This does not ignore the fact that agreeing enhanced services can be a lot more difficult in other areas. (It can be worthwhile, however, to compare where we are now in terms of enhanced services to where we were, say, two years ago.)

Secondly, having them here can be useful as a reference tool to see what other areas have agreed as service specifications for various enhanced services. The list is by no means exhaustive (you can obtain a fuller list from the GPC office). There is no point reinventing the wheel; instead you can spend your time improving or adapting.

Thirdly, seeing prices previously agreed for various services helps you to judge the market and pitch your bid. I would always suggest, though, that you do your individual costs and profit expectations separately first, and then use these and other established enhanced services as a gauge.

Fourthly, some PCOs are trying to reinterpret what are essential services and what are enhanced services. They are trying to say that if you provided a service before the new contract, it is essential work. Tosh! Essential work is defined in the regulations and no individual PCO, or group of PCOs for that matter, can redefine what is in or out. Basically, if I get paid for giving goserelin injections, then it is an enhanced service by definition.

As I have said, the list is not exhaustive. There are numerous other examples of different services, or similar services delivered in different ways and to different standards. Inclusion of a service on the list does not represent my endorsement in terms of the specification or costing. The aim is simply to show what has been done, what other GPs and LMCs have accepted and what is getting paid.

APPENDIX 1

AGREEING ENHANCED SERVICE FLOORS: GPC GUIDANCE FOR LMCs

GPC

General Practitioners Committee

BMA

The GPC has been asked on many occasions to produce a definitive list of what constitutes essential and enhanced services under the new contract in order to facilitate LMCs' negotiations with PCOs. We have resisted doing so because we believe that it is not possible to produce a list that is comprehensive and unarguable in every situation. There will always be local exceptions that national guidance could not cover, which LMCs should be free to agree if they believe they are appropriate in their area. However, the newly formed Enhanced Services Subgroup has been able to draw up a list that reflects the results of local negotiations between LMCs and PCOs on enhanced services across the UK in 2004/05 – this can be found at **Appendix 2**. LMCs should read the list in conjunction with the short paper 'Enhanced Services: how to tell what they are and whether or not they count towards the floor' found at **Appendix 3**.

The list has been divided into three broad categories: services that are enhanced services that can legitimately count towards the enhanced services floor (ESF), services that either are or are not enhanced services, but cannot count towards the ESF and services that, depending on local arrangements, the inclusion of in the ESF varies.

LMCs should bear in mind that the *can* section includes services that have been negotiated somewhere in the UK, but that it is unlikely that an LMC necessarily will be able to negotiate all of these services in their area. Where activity appears here as an enhanced service, it does not necessarily follow that the Subgroup considers this the best way to provide the service. If GPs do the work, they must be funded and the enhanced services floor is the appropriate mechanism for this. However, some of the activities may be best carried out by acute or community trusts. As regards those enhanced services, which will clearly result in a transfer of work from current hospital provision (e.g. some GPwSIs, diagnostics), they should be funded from the hospital commissioning budget and not from the ESF. LMCs should resist re-badging of services that historically have been funded through and provided by the secondary sector.

The *varies* section exists as a result of an example where historical, local factors mean that what in most areas would not count towards the enhanced services floor, in some areas does.

Although such a list can be neither definitive nor exhaustive, this does represent the authoritative view of the GPC on the enhanced services that have emerged to date that either can or cannot count towards the ESF.

We hope that this document will assist LMCs in their discussions with PCOs on ESF proposals in the run up to year end on 31 March 2005 and thereafter.

Every effort should be made to reach agreement by negotiation between the LMC and the PCO. Where, despite this, local disagreement on enhanced services and use of the spending floor persists, details of the dispute should be sent via the GPC secretariat LMC Liaison Officer to the Enhanced Services Subgroup for comment and/or action as appropriate. [Full terms of reference and membership of the Subgroup can be found at **Appendix 4**.] If the case remains unresolved, the issue can be submitted for consideration by the Implementation Co-ordination Group (ICG) of the Health Departments, the NHS Confederation and the GPC for final direction.

Brian Balmer
Joint Chairman
Enhanced Services Subgroup

Chaand Nagpaul
Joint Chairman
Enhanced Services Subgroup

February 2005

APPENDIX 2

ENHANCED SERVICE FLOOR LIST

GPC

General Practitioners
Committee

BMA

Enhanced services that can count towards the ESF:

1. All DESs and NESs
2. Nursing/residential homes
   Includes the enhanced element of care only
3. Refugees and asylum seekers
4. Prescribing and monitoring drugs not mentioned in the 'near-patient testing' NES
   Includes amiodarone, gold and sulphasalazine, lithium, etc
5. Initiation of secondary care drugs
   Includes insulin and initial monitoring under shared-care agreements such as depot psychotropics, Ritalin and alcohol dependency prescribing
   Note that 'shared care' must be genuine and not merely on the instruction of a consultant
6. Suture removals
   Note where there is a specific LES
7. Dressings post operation/leg ulcers
   Note where there is a specific LES
8. Minor/moderate surgery
   Includes vasectomy, sigmoidoscopy, carpal tunnel release, ingrowing toenails, etc
9. GPwSI (community)
   Includes dermatology, psychosexual counselling, allergy, genetic counselling, joint injections, vasectomy, urology, heart failure, gynaecology and podiatry
   Why? If the GPwSI is working in the community and providing enhanced community GMS, this can count towards the ESF. In addition, to count towards the ESF, the referral pathway should be GP to GPwSI and not via secondary care
10. Contraceptive implants/fittings
    Includes Proscar, Implanon, Depo-Provera, etc
    Why? These implants are not part of ordinary primary medical services as they require special training and technique
11. Other implants/injections
    Includes Zoladex, etc
12. Information collecting for PCO
    Includes waiting list validation

13. Unscheduled immunisations/vaccinations
    Includes MMR to students, hepatitis B for occupational health reasons, etc
14. Early morning/evening/weekend surgeries if done by practices at PCO request and funded by same
    Does not include emergency work
15. More specialised chronic disease care schemes (GPwSI type)
16. Pre-operative assessments requested by the hospital
    Includes MRSA screening
17. Phlebotomy that is not an essential part of GMS
    Includes blood tests as requested by the hospital and/or outpatients department
18. 24-hour blood pressure monitoring
19. Cardiac event monitoring (24-hour ECGs)
20. Routine neonatal checks following early discharge or home birth
21. Audiology screening
22. Glaucoma screening
23. Teenage sexual health drop-in clinics
24. Obesity/weight management service
25. Counselling
    Includes contestable service provided either by an independent organisation in the community and available to all GP patients and/or provided within surgeries
26. ECGs on external initiation
    Includes routine ECG for hypertension, palpitations or chest pain
27. Ring pessary insertion and changes
28. Patients with learning disabilities
29. Hospital transport/ambulance organisation

Services that either are or are not enhanced services, but cannot count towards the ESF:
1. GPwSI (hospital)
   Why not? If a GPwSI is working as a clinical assistant/staff grade in a routine outpatient clinic, this cannot count towards the ESF, which includes a GPwSI service based in the community
2. Therapies
   Such as physiotherapy, etc
   Why not? In most cases, this is the re-provision of secondary care in GP surgeries or community health settings and is therefore not an enhanced service (and cannot count towards the ESF). However, where a new, additional service for patients, which can be tendered for by GMS and PMS contractors, is established, this would be an enhanced service
3. Pharmacy work
   Such as pharmacy advisors
4. Dental work
5. Secondary care carried out in the community
   Such as work done by consultants and specialist nurses
6. Community hospital current contacts
   Unless there is, for example, a new minor injury unit
7. Normal out-of-hours work

8. Prescribing incentive schemes
   Why not? They are not medical or patient services; they are not contestable; they are not provided *to* patients and the schemes have never been funded by GMS money (or hospital money), but from completely separate prescribing budgets
9. PRIMIS facilitator
10. Citizens Advice workers (practice based)
    Why not? This is not an enhanced service because it is a social, not clinical, service nor is it the provision of patient care
11. Evercare nursing model and community matrons
12. Medical certificates for patients who have been in hospital

Services that, depending on local arrangements, the inclusion of in the ESF varies:
1. Mental health workers

APPENDIX 3

ENHANCED SERVICES: HOW TO TELL WHAT THEY ARE AND WHETHER OR NOT THEY COUNT TOWARDS THE FLOOR

GPC

General Practitioners
Committee

The GMS contract guidance document *Delivering Investment in General Practice: Implementing the New Contract* states the following in relation to the definition of enhanced services:

"2.77 PCTs will be placed under a duty through directions to commission all six current Directed Enhanced Services (DES) to meet the needs of their population. In line with paragraph 2.13 of *Investing in General Practice*, the Contract Regulations define enhanced services as follows:

'medical services other than essential services, additional services or out of hours services; or essential services, additional services or out of hours services or an element of such a service that a contractor agrees under the contract to provide in accordance with specifications set out in a plan, which requires of the contractor an enhanced level of service provision to that which it needs generally to provide in relation to that service or element of service.'

The Contract Regulations allow the medical services to be of any type, in any setting, and to extend beyond the scope of primary medical services. There is no legal constraint as to what types of NHS medical services a PCT can commission through the four provider routes described in section A of this chapter. This will give PCTs a broad ability to develop more integrated services across the primary, secondary and acute sectors.

2.78 **However, for the purposes of financial monitoring, the definition of enhanced services is drawn more tightly than the legal definition.** PCTs will be notified of their enhanced services expenditure floor level in the January 2004 allocations, which they will be expected to meet but can exceed. PCTs will need to consider carefully what constitutes an enhanced service for the purpose of accurate financial monitoring. This will be undertaken at national level by the joint BMA/NHS Confederation/Health Departments Technical Steering Committee. Whilst a precise national definition would not be sufficiently sensitive to local issues, PCTs and contractors should bear in mind that, generally speaking, the following spend would count towards the floor:

(i)   Commissioning, or direct PCT provision, of Directed, National or Locally Enhanced Services from any provider, not just GMS and PMS contractors

(ii)   Practitioners With a Special Interest (PWSIs) **except in relation to essential or additional services**

(iii) The **plus element** of PMS Plus and the **specialist element** of specialist PMS arrangements

(iv)   Local primary medical care incentive schemes commissioned from GMS or PMS providers

(v)   If the PCT proposed, for example, to re-commission a service that had previously been placed with an NHS trust it would count towards the floor, regardless of the outcome of the contest, but only providing that:

(a)   **It was contestable for GMS and PMS contractors**

(b)   **It is a service that might reasonably be provided by GMS and PMS contractors,** for example because looking across the UK there are other such contractors delivering similar services."

The following is a simple checklist of questions to which if the answer is NO, then the service does not count towards the Enhanced Services Floor (ESF):

1. **Does it provide a higher level or specialisation of care to patients?**
2. **Is it contestable by GPs?**
3. **Can it reasonably be provided by GPs?**

The following questions, if answered YES, would again suggest that the proposed service is NOT an enhanced service that counts towards the ESF:

1. **Does it provide essential or additional services to patients?**
2. **Is it spend on primary care services funded through other routes?**
3. **Is it spend on essential services, e.g. premises, greenfield sites?**
4. **Is it funding the provision of out-of-hours services?**
5. **Is it baseline spend for services provided by trusts, e.g. accident and emergency, existing services provided by GPs in community hospitals or as clinical assistants, and provided under an existing contract?**

The LMC should be consulted about the proposed level of spend and the PCO should seek to obtain LMC agreement that the proposed services count within the above definition for financial monitoring purposes. Where there is a dispute over what counts towards the floor, the LMC and PCO should seek to resolve this locally in the first instance.

PCOs will be under a **legal obligation** to commission services for violent patients (from 1 February 2004), influenza immunisations, and minor surgery (both from 1 April 2004). These can be commissioned from any provider, or the PCO can provide the service itself. However, it is likely that PCOs will in most instances want to commission these services from the patients' own GMS and PMS contractors, to ensure continuity of care.

The PCO commissions enhanced services as primary medical services; they only become GMS services when they are provided as part of a GMS contract. The PCO has discretion to draw up specifications on the basis of local need and it can also decide when it wants to commission most enhanced services.

For example, a PCO could choose to commission minor surgery from a PMS or commercial contractor using a different specification and at a different price from the GMS NES specification. Nonetheless, PCOs may wish to be guided by the twelve GMS NES specifications as detailed in the 'Supporting Documentation' (i.e. second, thicker blue book). GMS contractors may expect, and may only be willing, to offer enhanced services on the basis of the GMS NES specifications and prices.

Some PMS practices may already be funded for some enhanced service activity within their existing contracts and the PCO may choose to review these.

Commissioning decisions are entirely a matter for local negotiation (and the contract dispute resolution procedure described in chapter 6 does not apply); PCOs will want to make commissioning decisions on the basis of quality, accessibility, choice, and value for money. PCOs will also want to consider the duration of such contracts.

APPENDIX 4

ENHANCED SERVICES SUBGROUP OF THE GPC's PRIMARY CARE DEVELOPMENT SUBCOMMITTEE

GPC

General Practitioners
Committee

Terms of reference
* To comment on enhanced services spending floor proposals from PCOs as and when necessary at the request of LMCs (as routed via the LMC Liaison Officer)
* To comment on definitions of essential and enhanced services as and when necessary at the request of LMCs (as routed via the LMC Liaison Officer)
* To recommend to the GPC UK negotiators where a dispute between an LMC and PCO regarding the enhanced services spending floor should be considered by the Implementation Coordination Group (ICG)
* To collect/disseminate examples of good practice from/to LMCs
* To build a library of agreed LES specifications for dissemination among LMCs

Membership
Joint chairmen
Brian Balmer — Chief Executive of North and South Essex LMCs (and GPC member)
Chaand Nagpaul — Chairman of the GPC's Primary Care Development Subcommittee

GPC negotiators
Andrew Dearden — Chairman of GPC Wales
Richard Vautrey — Medical Secretary of Leeds LMC

LMC representatives
Andrew Green — Chairman of East Yorkshire LMC
Peter Jolliffe — Chief Officer of Devon LMCs

Primary Care Development Subcommittee
Helena McKeown
Sally Nelson — Director of Public Health, South Wiltshire PCT
Simon Poole — Chairman of Cambridgeshire LMC
Peter Swinyard

CRITERIA FOR LOCAL ENHANCED SERVICES

When you design an LES it may be helpful to use the NES specifications as a template. The various sections of the terms and conditions may be:

1. Clinical evidence and data to determine the design, size and scope of service provision

2. Service protocols

3. Developing and maintaining a register of patients

4. Determining the service to be delivered

5. Specifying the skills required to deliver the service or using an appraisal mechanism to ensure ongoing service standards

6. Providing a personal health and record plan

7. Ensuring that the care given is recorded in the lifelong GP-held patient record

8. Communication between the GP provider and the patient's GP, if they are not part of the same practice

9. Involving, where appropriate, carers and support workers/services

10. Ensuring regular liaison, where appropriate, with carers and support workers/social services

11. Developing screening procedures to improve clinical outcomes, including medication reviews

12. Providing patient reference material

13. Continuing professional development

14. Annual review and audit of the service

15. Developing appropriate quality standards

16. Special training

17. Accreditation

18. Additional resources

19. Infrastructure/costs, e.g. staff time, equipment, etc.

20. General contract review

APPENDIX 6
HOW TO COST A LOCAL ENHANCED SERVICE

Costs incurred in providing the service:

1. Practice staff (remember to include all costs, e.g. wages, national insurance, pension contributions, etc.)

New clinical staff, e.g. healthcare assistant   ----------------------

Additional administrative staff hours   ----------------------

Additional administrative staff training   ----------------------

New nurse/nurse practitioner staff cost   ----------------------

Additional current nurse/nurse practitioner hours   ----------------------

Additional current nurse/nurse practitioner training   ----------------------

Additional practice staff medico-legal cover   ----------------------

2. Equipment

New equipment needed   ----------------------

Additional training needed in using equipment   ----------------------

Running costs of equipment, e.g. consumables   ----------------------

Maintenance of equipment, e.g. annual calibration
  tests   ----------------------

Additional insurance/contract costs for equipment   ----------------------

3. Premises

Additional room/space needed   ----------------------

Running costs, e.g. electricity, heating   ----------------------

Additional decoration/use costs   ----------------------

Consumables   ----------------------

4. Doctors

Additional doctor hours   ----------------------

Additional/ongoing doctor training:

   – Costs of training   ----------------------

   – Locum/backfill costs   ----------------------

Additional legal cover costs   ----------------------

Total cost   ----------------------

APPENDIX 7
HOW TO CALCULATE THE PROFIT ELEMENT OF A CONTRACT

Option 1

Use a standard percentage of the total contract price

- For example, the Red Book expenses:earnings ratio was around 60:40
- So costs of £60 would mean a profit level of £40 = total costs of £100
- Using this method profit = 66% of costs

Option 2

Use identifiable doctor hours

- Each practice will need to set its own rate for doctor hours

Option 3

Decide the amount you want to earn after costs

- This may reflect workload, intensity, etc.

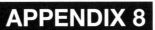
APPENDIX 8
LIST OF LOCAL ENHANCED SERVICES HELD AT THE GPC OFFICES

24-hour ambulatory blood pressure monitoring
Adur, Arun and Worthing PCT (with pricing)

Anticoagulation monitoring
Erewash PCT (with pricing)

Asylum seekers
Adur, Arun and Worthing PCT (with pricing)
Hastings and St Leonards PCT (with pricing)
Oxford PCT (with pricing)

Assisted conception
Southern Derbyshire PCT (without pricing)

Bank holiday cover
Surrey Heath and Woking PCT (without pricing)

Brief health promotion interventions in primary care
Adur, Arun and Worthing PCT (with pricing)

Chronic disease management
Bexhill and Rother PCT (with pricing)

Chronic obstructive pulmonary disease
Doncaster East PCT (with pricing)

Clinical governance administrative support
Doncaster central PCT (with pricing)

Continuation of services
Hambleton and Richmondshire PCT (with pricing)

Contraceptive implant fitting and removal
Brighton and Hove City PCT (with pricing)
Derbyshire Dales and South Derbyshire PCT (with pricing)
Erewash PCT (with pricing)
Hastings and St Leonards PCT (with pricing)

Child protection for GP practices
Brighton and Hove City PCT (with pricing)

Depot antipsychotic drugs
Southern Derbyshire PCT (without pricing)

Depot hormone replacement therapy
Southern Derbyshire PCT (without pricing)

Diabetes management
Doncaster East PCT (with pricing)
East Surrey PCT (with pricing)
Hastings and St Leonards PCT (with pricing)
Unclear which practice (under Brighton and Hove PCT) (with pricing)

Diabetic retinopathy
Bexhill and Rother PCT (with pricing)

Drug misuse
Adur, Arun and Worthing PCT (with pricing)
Powys LHB (with pricing)

Drug monitoring
Adur, Arun and Worthing PCT (with pricing)

Electrocardiograph recording
Selby and York PCT (with pricing)

Enhanced single-dose vaccinations
Doncaster West PCT (with pricing)

Enhanced treatment room support: levels 1 and 2
Unclear which PCT, under Doncaster (without pricing)

Extended minor surgery (injections above DES activity; invasive procedures above DES activity)
Greater Derby and Central Derby PCTs (with pricing)

Extended services to nursing homes
Rhondda Cynon Taff region (with pricing)

Follow up of prostate cancer
Newcastle PCT (with pricing)

GP services to nursing homes
North Eastern Derbyshire PCT (with pricing)

Growth hormone
Southern Derbyshire PCT (no pricing)

Heart failure
Bexhill and Rother PCT (with pricing)

Healthy choices
Doncaster East PCT (with pricing)

Hepatitis B vaccination
Unclear which PCT, under Doncaster (with pricing)

HIV
Brighton and Hove City PCT (with pricing)

Immediate and first-response care
Unclear which PCT (under Brighton and Hove PCT file) (with pricing)

Improved access to GMS
Unclear which PCT (under Doncaster PCT) (some pricing information)

Influenza vaccination campaign 2004
Selby and York PCT (with pricing)

Influenza vaccination bonus payments
Erewash PCT (with pricing)

Insulin initiation
Derbyshire Dales and South Derbyshire PCT (with pricing)

Learning disability
Doncaster East PCT (with pricing)
Selby and York PCT (with pricing)

Leg ulcers
Brighton and Hove City PCT (with pricing)

Major depression: diagnosis and treatment
Brighton and Hove City PCT (with pricing)

Medical cover for 'Archways' (an intermediate care unit)
Selby and York PCT (with pricing)

Minor injuries service
Bexhill and Rother PCT (with pricing)
Greater Derby and Central Derby PCTs (with pricing)
Hambleton and Richmondshire PCT (with pricing)

Minor surgery
Hastings and St Leonards PCT (with pricing)

MMR catch up
Brighton and Hove City PCT (with pricing)
Greater Derby and Central Derby PCTs (with pricing)

MMR for university students
Eastbourne Downs PCT (with pricing)

Mumps vaccination
Hambleton and Richmondshire PCT (with pricing)
Liverpool PCTs (with pricing)
Walsall PCT (with pricing)

Near-patient testing for shared-care drugs
Derbyshire Dales and South Derbyshire PCT (with pricing)
Erewash PCT (with pricing)
Greater Derby and Central Derby PCTs (with pricing)

'New entrant' (immigrant) services
Greater Derby and Central Derby PCTs (with pricing)

Nursing homes
Hambleton and Richmondshire PCT (with pricing)

Palliative care
Brighton and Hove City PCT (with pricing)

Personality disorder
Brighton and Hove City PCT (with pricing)

Pharmacist support
Doncaster Central PCT (with pricing)

Phlebotomy
Adur, Arun and Worthing PCT (with pricing)
Brighton and Hove City PCT (with pricing)
Selby and York PCT (with pricing)

Pneumococcal immunisation
Woking area PCT (with pricing)

Pregnancy testing for young people
Adur, Arun and Worthing PCT (with pricing)

Provision of gonadorelin analogue treatments under shared-care guidelines
Derbyshire Dales and South Derbyshire PCT (with pricing)
Greater Derby and Central Derby PCTs (with pricing)

Public health vaccinations
Unclear which PCT (in North Yorkshire) (with pricing)

Saturday service
East Surrey PCT (with pricing)

Shared prescribing
Richmond and Twickenham (draft form, no pricing details)

Sigmoidoscopy
Selby and York PCT (with pricing for one group practice only)

Smoking cessation
Erewash PCT (with pricing)
Hastings and St Leonards PCT (with pricing)
Southern Derbyshire (with no pricing)
Unclear which PCT (in North Yorkshire) (with pricing)
Western Sussex PCT (with pricing)

Specialist community dermatology
Brighton and Hove City PCT (with pricing)

Student health
Selby and York PCT (with pricing for one practice only)

Substance misuser services
Derbyshire Dales and South Derbyshire PCT (with pricing)

Teenage and young person's sexual health
Brighton and Hove City PCT (with pricing)

University health centre, minor injuries and immunisations
Sussex university, unclear which PCT (no pricing)

Vaccinations/immunisations for public health purposes
Derbyshire Dales and South Derbyshire PCT (with pricing)

Weight management
Unclear which trust, under 'Brighton and Hove PCT' (no pricing)

Women's refuge services
Derbyshire Dales and South Derbyshire PCT (with pricing)

Wound care and suture removal
Selby and York PCT (with pricing)

Wound closure
Brighton and Hove City PCT (with pricing)

Young people
Doncaster East PCT (with pricing)

Zoladex
Southern Derbyshire PCT (no pricing)

Basket LES

Adur, Arun and Worthing PCT (with pricing examples)
- Catheter, ulcer, and wound care in nursing homes
- Inspecting and/or syringing ears at the request of the hospital
- Removal of post-operative sutures
- Triage and advice for minor injuries
- Vault smears
- Signing homely remedy forms
- Booking transport for patients

Eastbourne Downs PCT (with draft pricing)
- Secondary post-operative care, including removal of sutures and clips and attention to wound dressings
- Complex dressing procedures, such as triple-layer dressings for chronic venous ulceration
- Phlebotomy (within the practice and domiciliary)
- Ordering or undertaking investigations for patients under hospital care (e.g. as identified under NESs for near-patient testing and INR monitoring)
- Prescribing while hospital care continues (e.g. as identified under NESs for near-patient testing and INR monitoring) to be extended to include treatments such as complex rheumatological, chemotherapeutic and long-acting drugs given by injections, e.g. neuroleptics and luteinising hormone releasing hormone analogues
- Insertion of hormone implants
- Care for patients in nursing homes, residential homes and frail elderly at home
- Treatment of minor injuries (e.g. laceration capable of simple closure, bruises, superficial burns, minor head injuries with no loss of consciousness)
- Aural care
- *Helicobacter pylori* testing
- Catheter and stoma care (community only)
- Arranging patient transport
- Pregnancy testing, where immediately necessary for diagnostic purposes
- Prescribing drugs that Midland Therapeutic Review and Advisory Committee defines as appropriate for shared-care protocols as of 31 March 2004, e.g. methylphenidate, erythropoietin, gosarelin, leuprorelin, drugs for erectile dysfunction
- Emergency phlebotomy, where immediately necessary for diagnostic purposes
- Twelve-lead ECGs
- Pre-employment vaccination for healthcare professionals
- Three-year cervical smear checks
- Mental health and learning disability care for which GP contractors would not normally have the specialist skills to accept full responsibility
- Removal of foreign bodies from eyes, ears and nose
- Audiometry
- Secondary care or specialist clinical sampling (including phlebotomy and RheMOS testing)
- Ambulatory blood pressure monitoring
- Administration of injectable drugs

Guildford and Waverley PCT (with pricing)
'Complementary services'
- Post-operative services
- Investigations
- Phlebotomy
- Providing information
- Skin ulcers

Selby and York (with pricing)
'Supplementary medical services'
- Requests to arrange ambulance transportation for patients attending hospital and/or community services
- Postnatal checks undertaken by GPs, including postnatal hip checks and routine postnatal checks for patients with postvaginal or uncomplicated caesarean section
- Administration of subcutaneous depot injections, e.g. gosarelin
- Administration of depot neuroleptics
- Blood sampling for clozapine monitoring
- Monitoring of drugs provided through shared-care arrangements

Western Sussex PCT (with pricing)
This service will include, but not be limited to, the following services:
- Post-operative suture removal
- Treatment room procedures including dressing of ulcers, ear syringing
- Leuprorelin and gosarelin injections
- Pre-referral assessments
- Provision of audit and referral information as required by the PCT

West Hull PCT (with pricing)
- Requests for phlebotomy in general practice as a consequence of a referral to or ongoing care by hospital services, where it is inconvenient or undesirable for the patient to attend hospital
- Requests for removal of sutures, where the operation was carried out outside general practice as a consequence of a referral to or ongoing care by hospital services, where it is inconvenient or undesirable for the patient to attend hospital
- Requests to arrange ambulance transportation for patients attending hospital and/or community services as a consequence of a referral to or ongoing care, where the local ambulance service is unable to provide a direct service to patients or where the patient is unable to make a direct request
- Providing information to screening services or other public health initiatives commissioned by a PCT

APPENDIX 9

SOUTH WILTSHIRE PCT SERVICE LEVEL AGREEMENT FOR LOCAL ENHANCED SERVICE: INITIATION OF INSULIN IN TYPE 2 DIABETES

Contents
- Financial details
- Service aims
- Criteria
- Ongoing measurement and evaluation

Financial details
In 2003/4 the provision of this local enhanced service will be £75 per patient for conversion initiated by the patient's own GP and practice nurse. There will also be an annual retainer of £800 to cover training and audit requirements.

Service aims
It is well documented that the incidence of type 2 diabetes is increasing rapidly, and that more patients with type 2 diabetes are being started on insulin earlier than before. *Shifting the Balance of Power*, the *National Service Framework for Diabetes* delivery strategy and the Quality and Outcomes Framework encourage individual practices to deliver structured diabetes care and take on more of the uncomplicated diabetes management. The aim of this enhanced service is therefore to:
- Enhance continuity of care
- Ensure the service to the patient is convenient and timely
- Facilitate keeping the person with diabetes in primary care.

Patients with more complex needs will continue to be referred to the PCT specialist diabetes service.

Criteria
All practices are expected to provide essential and those additional services they are contracted to provide to all their patients. This enhanced service specification outlines the more specialised services to be provided. The specification of this service is designed to cover the enhanced aspects of clinical care of the patient, all of which are beyond the scope of essential services. No part of the specification by commission, omission or implication defines or redefines essential or additional services.

The practice taking on this local enhanced service will:

(i)   Register
Practices should maintain an up-to-date register of all patients converted to insulin in the practice.

(ii)   Call and recall
To ensure the systematic recall of all patients who have undergone insulin conversion and that there are systems in place for ensuring regular contact during initial stages for dose adjustment.

(iii) Patient education
To ensure that all people converted to insulin (and/or their carers) receive appropriate education and advice on the management of insulin-treated diabetes. This should include written information.

(iv)   Professional links
To work together with other healthcare professionals. Including formal ongoing mentoring from the specialist diabetes service.

(v)   Training
Each practice must ensure that staff providing any aspect of care under this scheme do so in accordance with the training provided by the specialist diabetes service.

Ongoing measurement and evaluation
The practice should conduct an annual review to include:

(a) Feedback from staff and diabetic patients

(b) An audit of the service including any problems experienced

(c) Data on the length and number of consultations required.

A report on this review should be submitted to the primary care development manager at South Wiltshire PCT highlighting recommendations/action planned for the next year.

APPENDIX 10

SOUTH WILTSHIRE PCT SERVICE LEVEL AGREEMENT FOR LOCAL ENHANCED SERVICE: EXAMINATION OF THE NEWBORN BABY

Contents
- Financial details
- Service aims
- Criteria
- Ongoing measurement and evaluation

Financial details
This agreement is to cover the 12 months commencing 1 April 2005. For each check performed within the target period the practice is entitled to £53.27.

Service aims
All practices are expected to provide essential and those additional services they are contracted to provide to all their patients. No part of the specification by commission, omission or implication defines or redefines essential or additional services. The initial examination of the newborn commences the Department of Health infant health surveillance programme. It is included in the national specification for intra-partum care so is not seen as part of the child surveillance additional service.

The purpose of the first examination of the newborn baby is to undertake a full assessment to identify any congenital abnormalities that may or may not have been diagnosed during fetal development or those related to transition to newborn life and future development. In addition, this assessment provides an opportunity to provide health and social education advice to parents.

Ideally the neonatal first examination should be undertaken within 72 hours (Universal Child Health Surveillance Programme for Wiltshire, 2002). The check should, however, be done within 24 hours of birth when it does not occur over a weekend or bank holiday. It should normally be performed before discharge from hospital for hospital births, thus being carried out within the optimal period and minimising length of stay for normal healthy babies. This should be undertaken in the community for home births.

A neonatal examination by a skilled GP or midwife is appropriate for all healthy, normal term newborn babies born after 37 completed weeks. Exceptions to this are:
- Any maternal disease where it may impact on the neonate
- Any obvious congenital abnormality

- Any apparent trauma (chignon on baby's head following Ventouse extraction, fractured clavicle and any cuts following fetal scalp application) other than superficial
- Any neonate who required medical input prior to the first check being performed
- Any neonates with jaundice occurring within 24 hours
- Any baby who required red star observations.

Any of the above babies should have the first examination undertaken by a paediatrician.

Criteria
This local enhanced service will fund:
- **Services** – the examination described in appendix 1 [note: not included here], including referral on where appropriate, will be provided by a member of practice staff
- **Clinical procedures** – to ensure that all clinical information related to the LES is recorded in the patient's own GP held lifelong record
- **Record keeping** – to maintain adequate records of the performance and result of the service provided, incorporating information related to any significant events
- **Audit** – to carry out clinical audit of the care of patients, including untoward incidents
- **Training** – each practice must ensure that all staff involved in providing any aspect of care under this scheme have the necessary training and skills to do so.

Ongoing measurement and evaluation
All practices involved in this scheme should perform an annual review of the service provided against the specification outlined above and the quality of care received by the relevant patients.

APPENDIX 11
SOUTH WILTSHIRE PCT SERVICE LEVEL AGREEMENT FOR LOCAL ENHANCED SERVICE: CONTRACEPTIVE IMPLANTS

Contents
- Financial details
- Service aims
- Criteria
- Ongoing measurement and evaluation

Financial details
This agreement is to cover the 12 months commencing 1 April 2005. In 2005/6 each practice contracted to provide the contraceptive implant service will receive a £25 insertion fee and £30 removal fee per patient.

Service aims
All practices are expected to provide essential and those additional services they are contracted to provide to all their patients. No part of the specification by commission, omission or implication defines or redefines essential or additional services.

Evidence shows that:
- The use of contraceptive implants has doubled since 2000, with over 10,000 implants being fitted in 2003
- Contraceptive implants provide excellent contraceptive protection over a long period. Implanon, which is the only contraceptive implant currently licensed in the UK, is reported to have a Pearl Index of 0.0 (95% CI 0.00–0.09).
- Implants are one of two areas of contraceptive provision with relatively high levels of litigation. The most important factor influencing the incidence of problems relating to insertion and removal is the competence of the professional inserting the device
- High-quality information and advice influences client satisfaction and continuation rates with long-acting methods of contraception
- Implant fitting and removal are not undertaken by all clinical practitioners in general practices and maintaining expertise in fitting and removal can be difficult and requires commitment from the practitioner.

The aims of this service are to:
- Ensure that the full range of contraceptive options is provided by practices to patients
- Increase the availability of contraceptive implants through primary care.

Criteria

This locally enhanced service will fund:
- **Fitting, monitoring, checking and removal of contraceptive implants** licensed for use in the UK, as appropriate according to product guidelines
- **Production of an up-to-date register of patients fitted with a contraceptive implant.** This will include all patients fitted with a contraceptive implant and the device fitted. This is to be used for audit purposes, and to enable these patients to be targeted for healthcare checks
- **Practitioners to undertake regular continual professional development**
- **Provision of adequate equipment.** Certain special equipment is required for implant fitting and removal. This includes an appropriate room fitted with a couch and with adequate space and equipment for resuscitation. A variety of removal forceps, and facility for local anaesthesia provision also need to be available. This specification also includes the provision of sterile surgical instruments and other consumables. An appropriately trained assistant also needs to be present to support the patient and assist the clinician during the procedure
- **The provision of condoms to prevent infection and public health information on safer sex practices**
- **Sexual history taking.** To ensure that the contraceptive implant is the most appropriate method of contraception based on medical evidence, clinical guidelines, sexual history and practice and risk assessment
- **Risk assessment.** To assess the need for sexually transmitted infection (STI) or HIV testing prior to recommending the contraceptive implant
- **Assessment and follow up.** Routine annual checks are not required. However, arrangements should be in place to review patients experiencing problems in a timely fashion. Arrangements should be in place to ensure timely access for women requesting removal of the implant for any reason including problems or at expiry of device. The implant should be removed or replaced within three years
- **Provision of information.** Appropriate verbal and written information about all contraceptive options should be provided at the time of counselling to ensure informed choice. Understanding regarding implant use should be reinforced at fitting with information on effectiveness, duration of use, side-effects and those symptoms that require urgent assessment
- **Production of an appropriate clinical record.** Adequate recording should be made regarding the patient's clinical, reproductive and sexual history, the counselling process, the results of any STI screening, problems with insertion, the type and batch number of the implant, expiry date of the device and follow-up arrangements. If the patient is not registered with the provider of the LES, the provider must ensure that the patient's registered practice is given all appropriate clinical details for inclusion into the patient's notes after obtaining explicit consent from the patient.

Ongoing measurement and evaluation

Practitioners undertaking these procedures should have had appropriate training. This should be based on modern, authoritative medical opinion, for example, the current requirements set down by the Faculty of Family Planning and Reproductive Health Care (FFPRHC) for the letter of competence in subdermal implants or Royal College of Nursing (RCN) guidance on insertion and removal of subdermal implants together with RCN accreditation.

This involves a demonstration of skills involved in counselling for implants, knowledge of issues relevant to implant use, problem management and observation of insertion and removal followed by supervised insertion and removal of a minimum number of insertions and removals as specified by the FFPRHC/RCN (as appropriate), and assessment of competence by a faculty- or RCN-approved assessor. They should provide evidence of maintaining skills, for example by re-certifying according to FFPRHC/RCN regulations.

Clinicians who have previously provided services similar to the proposed enhanced service and who satisfy at appraisal and revalidation that they have such continuing medical experience, training and competence as is necessary to enable them to contract for the enhanced service (by being considered equivalent to the requirements set down by the FFPRHC/RCN) shall be deemed professionally qualified to do so.

All practices involved in this scheme should perform an annual review of the service provided against the specification outlined above and the quality of care received by the relevant patients. This should include:

- The number of patients fitted with a contraceptive implant
- Reasons for removal
- Complications or significant events.

SOUTH WILTSHIRE PCT SERVICE LEVEL AGREEMENT FOR LOCAL ENHANCED SERVICE: 'NO SCALPEL' VASECTOMIES

The following is the basis of a service agreement between South Wiltshire PCT and Dr X for the provision of 'no scalpel' vasectomies to patients of practices in South Wiltshire.

Service description
Dr X will provide no scalpel vasectomies in accordance with the terms of this agreement.

Quality standards and service conditions
The Practitioner
The procedures will be carried out by Dr X only. Specifically, he will not depute any procedure under this scheme to a locum, registrar or any other practitioner. Dr X is registered with the GMC and is insured by the Medical Practitioners Protection Scheme. Dr X will be responsible for ensuring that his skills are regularly updated.

Service location
The procedures will be carried out at the Y Surgery, Salisbury, Wiltshire.

Location facilities
The surgery has a bespoke room for minor surgery. An experienced registered general nurse, fully trained in minor surgery, will be on site and available when procedures are taking place and a trained healthcare assistant will assist Dr X during procedures. A high standard of infection control protocols are in place and these are compliant with national guidelines. Protocols must be available to the PCT for inspection, if so requested. It is the responsibility of Dr X to ensure that adequate and appropriate equipment is available for the procedures undertaken, including appropriate equipment for resuscitation.

Service administration
Appointments
Appointments may be made with Dr X by the patient's GP in writing, using the mail, hospital courier or fax. Appointments will be sent to the patient within three working days for the procedure to be carried out within 28 working days in all

cases. The patient will receive directions and other appropriate instructions. All appointments will be engaged within 15 minutes of the appointment time.

Information to the patient
All patients will receive a full explanation of treatment options and will give written consent to the procedure being carried out. The completed NHS consent forms should be filed in the patient's lifelong medical record. The patient will receive appropriate regional anaesthesia and, where appropriate, a short supply of post-operate analgesia. The patient will also receive verbal and, if appropriate, written instructions for post-operative care including sperm samples. The patient will be sent results by post when available.

Information to the patient's GP
Full details of the procedure carried out will be sent to the patient's GP the next working day. Histology and a copy of the letter sent to the patient will be sent to the patient's GP when available.

Record keeping
All procedures will be recorded by Dr X and kept at Y Surgery for 10 years. Dr X accepts responsibility for levying appropriate invoices to the PCT and for ensuring accuracy of payments.

Audit
Full records of all procedures will be maintained in such a way that aggregated data and details of individual are readily accessible. The service will be regularly audited to review:
- Clinical outcomes
- Rates of infection.

Clinical responsibilities
Dressings
The patient will have their wound dressed appropriately after the procedure, before returning home. Thereafter further dressings, removal of sutures and aftercare are the responsibility of the patient's GP.

Fitness to work
The patient will be advised on general activities and fitness to work. Certification for social security and statutory sick pay purposes is the responsibility of the patient's GP.

Referral
The patient's GP is responsible for providing a referral letter containing details of the condition to be treated, pertinent past medical history, medications and allergies.

Cessation of services
Either party may terminate this agreement, giving three months' notice in writing. In the event of the service ceasing to operate, this agreement shall be deemed to

have terminated. In these circumstances the provider shall refund to the PCT any sums paid in advance under this agreement, to be calculated on a pro-rata basis for the unexpired part of the financial year, having regard to non-recoverable costs incurred.

Included in the cost

Procedures are 'inclusive' in that they are flat rate payments for all that is needed for each procedure. Disposables, drugs, dressings, maintenance of equipment and salaries, etc are all provided for within the fixed-rate payment and no surcharges will be levied. All necessary equipment and consumables will be purchased by Dr X independently of the NHS GP service. All costs, however, relate to the procedure only; no liability is accepted for any postoperative costs, which will be included under the patient's GP NHS services.

Procedures

This contract is for the provision of no scalpel vasectomies and no other procedure.

Agreement period

This agreement will take the form of an annual contract. Either party may terminate this agreement giving three months' notice in writing. Modifications not affecting the contract value will be subject to at least one month's notice.

Financial arrangements

The maximum cost of the service to South Wiltshire PCT is set by practice. It will be at the discretion of the individual practice to refer patients to Dr X. The PCT will pay £160 per vasectomy on receipt of an invoice that states the number of procedures and each referring practice.

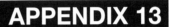

APPENDIX 13

BRO TAF LMC SERVICE LEVEL AGREEMENT FOR LOCAL ENHANCED SERVICE: EXTENDED SERVICES TO NURSING HOMES

Introduction

The purpose of this paper is to set out a model for a local enhanced service for the provision of GP services to high-dependency patients in nursing homes, and in the community.

The high-dependency patients to be included within the scope of this service are:
- Persons who are resident in registered nursing homes
- Persons who are very dependent in the community.

Definitions

Persons will be regarded as being:
- *Registered in a registered nursing home* provided it is a nursing home registered within the Rhondda Cynon Taff (RCT) region. It will not include persons registered in nursing homes outside the RCT region. It will not include persons receiving residential care under part 1 of the Registered Homes Act 1984, in a home that is registered to provide both nursing and residential care, i.e. a person not in a bed classified as a nursing bed
- *Very dependent in the community* requiring at least a weekly visit from the GP to reassess treatment or medication. They may possibly be receiving an intensive care package from other agencies, e.g. district nurse, house care, etc.

Service outline

GPs are required to provide the standard level of essential and additional services, as defined by the new GMS contract, to all nursing home patients registered with the GP practice.

The services required of GPs to be provided to persons being cared for under this local enhanced service, are to include the following.
- A mental and physical assessment on admission or within five working days of admission for all patients, including looking for signs of depression in the elderly physically incapacitated and physical complaints in those with mental and learning disabilities
- The regular review of the clinical management of all patients included under this local enhanced service. The GP should review the mental health, sensory

and nutritional status, advise on activity and preventative health measures, provide clinical summaries for each person covered, using the standard report format [Appendix 1 – note: this is not provided here]. Patients should be classified as follows, in agreement with nursing home staff, and the patient classification noted in the report [Appendix 1]:

- Level 1: Annual review
- Level 2: Quarterly review

- Regular review of medication, especially repeat medication at least six monthly. This should include blood screening and physical examination as appropriate on certain medication, i.e. warfarin, digoxin, thyroxine, enteral feeding requirements and palliative care arrangements by reviewing medication administration records and nursing care records or similar with nursing staff, in liaison as appropriate with a pharmacist to ensure their safe use
- Working with nursing and care staff to investigate, treat and manage incontinence through normal good practice and any protocols as and when agreed by the LMC
- Working with nursing and care staff when relevant to ensure tissue viability with a view to enabling older persons to remain as active as possible
- Team working and clinical risk assessment with appropriate staff in the nursing home, or, if applicable, in the community, through shared education or patient focused team building events as appropriate (e.g. through seminars, care conferences, etc).

Commissioning arrangements

Patient assessment reports should be made available for review to members of the LHB nursing and primary care team. A manual claims form should be made to the business services centre on LDS forms clearly indicating level 1 or level 2, in order to facilitate quarterly payments per patient.

Rates of payment are:
- Level 1 – £25.80 (per patient per annum)
- Level 2 – £151.29 (per patient per annum).

Schedules to Paragraph 14 of the Extended Statement of Fees and Allowances

Schedule 1 to Paragraph 14:
- Assessment of nursing care dependency form

Schedule 2 to Paragraph 14:
- Form ESNH/I
- Practitioner application form for payment of fees

Schedule 3 to Paragraph 14:
- Form ESNH/I/TR
- Temporary resident patient practitioner
- Application form for payment of fees

SPECIFICATION FOR A LOCAL ENHANCED SERVICE (WALES): GENERIC AGREEMENT FOR OFFERING IMMUNISATION DURING OUTBREAKS TO PATIENTS AT RISK

Introduction

The purpose of this document is to set out a model for a local enhanced service for immunisation of at-risk groups during outbreaks of infection.

Clinical guidance on immunisation promulgated by the Assembly will normally be based on the advice of the Joint Committee on Vaccination and Immunisation (JCVI). This is given in the most current version of the Green Book, or in the absence of such guidance produced by the Health Protection Agency or National Public Health Service for Wales. The need for local immunisation in response to a specific outbreak of vaccine-preventable disease will be identified by a Consultant in Communicable Disease Control (CCDC), or someone acting on their behalf.

All practices are expected to provide essential and those additional services they are contracted to provide to all their patients. This enhanced services specification outlines the more specialised services to be provided. The specification of this service is designed to cover enhanced aspects of clinical care of the patient, which go beyond the scope of essential services. No part of the specification by commission, omission or implication defines or redefines essential or additional services.

Aim

The purpose of the local enhanced service is to provide protection for individuals at increased risk of infection during a local outbreak of disease such as meningococcal meningitis, mumps, measles, etc.

Activation

This generic specification will be agreed in advance between LHBs and practices or other service provider, and Form A agreed between the CCDC and LHB at the time of an outbreak. Action should be taken by the individuals identified below, or their deputies.

When activated, Form A will provide details of the background to the outbreak, immunisation to be offered, the target group, vaccine supply and duration of the outbreak-specific agreement, converting this generic specification into a time-limited outbreak-specific agreement.

The LHB board should make arrangement to activate the LES without further prior reference to the board. This will allow flexibility and prompt action, which may be required on the same day an outbreak is identified. This could be achieved by delegating authority to one or more executive members.

The LES will come into effect only following agreement between the Chief Executive Officer of the LHB and the local CCDC in consultation with the local Public Health Director. The CCDC is responsible for seeking activation and providing details for Form A. The LHB will be responsible for informing practices of the outbreak-specific arrangements.

Where a practice has opted in advance not to participate in this LES, the LHB is responsible for making alternative arrangements to provide immunisation to those patients.

Eligibility

This will be dependent on the particular outbreak, which will be detailed in Form A. Payment arrangements will apply to all target patients who are immunised for the duration of the programme as set out in Form A.

How will the immunisation programme work?

Where practices are the preferred provider, practices will actively offer immunisation based on the details in Form A.

Individual GP practices will ensure each immunisation given under the LES is recorded on the individual's lifelong patient record, including passing information if providing immunisation on behalf of another practice. Practices will submit the usual unscheduled immunisations forms to the child health office for each child immunised to enable accurate monitoring of uptake.

No uptake target will be set. GPs should maximise uptake in the interests of patients. GPs are expected to take active steps to identify individuals in the target group and proactively offer immunisation. In all cases, the final decision as to who should be offered immunisation is a matter for the clinical judgement of the GP.

Some circumstances will require collaboration with the Community Child Health System (CCHS) office and use of the CCHS call and recall facility and, if so, this will be specified in Form A and practices will be informed.

In certain circumstances, to avoid overburdening practices, arrangements may be made with alternative service providers, such as trusts, to provide institution-based immunisation sessions. This may be necessary, for example, where entire schools require immunisation, or where immunisation is particularly urgent. In such circumstances, practices would provide support by immunising those who missed the immunisation sessions.

Existing arrangements will continue to apply in terms of obtaining supplies of vaccine, unless specified in Form A.

Pricing

LHBs should follow the national benchmark pricing for influenza and pneumococcal immunisations.

Form A

Outbreak name: _____

1. Specific outbreak details:

_____

_____

2. Immunisation to be offered (with reference to relevant national guidance):

_____

_____

3. Target group:

_____

4. Vaccine supply:

_____

5. Period within which vaccination should be offered:

_____

6. Activation and expiry date of this outbreak specific LES:

a. Activation date: /   /

b. Expiry date: /   /

SPECIFICATION FOR A LOCAL ENHANCED SERVICE (WALES): ADMINISTRATION OF GONADORELINS FOR PATIENTS WITH CARCINOMA OF THE PROSTATE

Introduction

All practices are expected to provide essential and those additional services they are contracted to provide to all their patients. This specification outlines the more specialised services to be provided. The specification of this service is designed to cover enhanced aspects of clinical care of the patient, which go beyond the scope of essential services. No part of the specification by commission, omission or implication defines or redefines essential or additional services.

Background

Gonadorelins are used primarily, though not exclusively, in the treatment of carcinoma of the prostate. There are a number of treatment regimes, which vary in the detail of their programme of administration and main purpose. Broadly they can be divided on the basis of the progress of the disease into advanced local disease and metastatic disease. The central use, however, remains the treatment of metastatic cancer of the prostate. Currently, it is estimated that over 95% of the prescriptions for gonadorelin analogues are written for carcinoma of the prostate.

Virtually all the prescriptions issued for injectable gonadorelins are written by GPs and most of these are also administered by GPs. In some practices an appropriately trained practice nurse will site the depot implants. The great majority of prescriptions are issued for Zoladex (generic name goselerin), which is administered subcutaneously into the anterior abdominal wall as a depot implant. Others are given subcutaneously or intramuscularly, depending on the indications and the preparation.

Different preparations are in place for treatment of carcinoma of the prostate, which are either injectable or implants. These are buserelin, goserelin, leuprorelin acetate and triptorelin. The majority of preparations for treatment of carcinoma of the prostate are goserelin implants or leuprorelin injections.

There are varying treatment models for administering gonadorelins to patients with carcinoma of the prostate dependent on the clinical management programme agreed for that patient.

Advice

This model service has been agreed between the Welsh Assembly Government and the General Practitioners Committee (Wales) for the administration of gonadorelins for patients with carcinoma of the prostate only.

LHBs should commission this from April 2005 and may wish to use the uplift in the enhanced services allocations for 2005/6 to meet the costs.

Aims
The administration of gonadorelins within primary care is designed to be an enhanced service in which:
- Patients with an established diagnosis and agreed treatment plan of carcinoma of the prostate, can undergo part of their treatment safely, effectively and conveniently close to their home
- There is much greater integration of primary and secondary care services and which recognises the increasing contribution that primary care can make in medical management and treatment of the hitherto predominantly hospital-based approach.

Service outline
It is a requirement of this national enhanced service that the contractor:

i.   **Provides a register** – practices will need to produce and maintain a valid up-to-date register of patients being treated as part of this enhanced service

ii.   **Demonstrates a call and recall system** – practices will need to ensure a systematic call and recall of patients on this register is taking place, and have in place the means to identify and follow up patients in default

iii. **Agrees a joint clinical management programme** – patients should be managed on the basis of individual treatment plans that will normally be drawn up by local consultants. Practices will be expected to follow these treatment plans unless there has been discussion and agreement with local consultants to modify them

iv.   **Supports the education of both newly diagnosed patients and those with established disease**. The secondary care oncology team will provide the main source of advice for both newly diagnosed patients and those with established disease. The practice will reinforce and supplement that advice where appropriate to do so

v.   **Provides an outline individual management plan** wherever possible to ensure that the patient has an outline individual management plan, which gives the reason for treatment, agreed treatment programme and the planned duration. This plan should be consistent with any agreed shared-care protocols

vi.   **Keeps records** – to maintain adequate records of the service provided, incorporating all known information relating to any significant events, e.g. adverse reactions, hospital admissions, and relevant deaths of which the practice has been notified

vii. **Ensures primary care staff training** – each practice must ensure that all staff involved in providing any aspect of care under this scheme have the necessary training and skills to do so. Practices should be able to demonstrate that they have in place a policy to cover staff training and maintenance of skills

viii. **Provides safe and suitable facilities for undertaking invasive procedures**
– LHBs should be satisfied that practices undertaking to provide the
Gonadorelin Administration Enhanced Service have adequate and
appropriate facilities and equipment comparable to those required for the
safe provision of any invasive procedure.

Untoward events

It is a condition of participation in this NES that practitioners will give
notification, within 72 hours of the information becoming known to him/her, to
the LHB clinical governance lead of all relevant significant adverse events,
emergency admissions or deaths of any patient treated under this service. This is
in addition to any statutory obligations.

Accreditation

Doctors will need to satisfy, at appraisal, that they have the necessary medical
experience, training and competence necessary to enable them to provide for a
safe and effective gonadorelin enhanced service.

Pricing

Given the different modes of administering gonadorelins for carcinoma of the
prostate, an annual fee has been set for 2005/6 for providing an individual
treatment package for patients as set out in the service outline of this specification.

The annual fees applicable are: all patients entering the scheme will attract an
annual fee of £100, which will be payable quarterly in arrears, provided that at
least one injection has been given in the relevant quarter. Existing patients, with
an established diagnosis of carcinoma of the prostate, who require continuation of
their gonadorelin treatment beyond 2005 will be regarded as new patients entering
the scheme and will attract an annual retention fee of £100, which is payable
quarterly in arrears, provided the patient has received at least one injection in the
relevant quarter.

APPENDIX 16

SPECIFICATION FOR A LOCAL ENHANCED SERVICE (WALES): CARE OF PEOPLE WITH LEARNING DISABILITIES

Introduction

All practices are expected to provide the essential and additional services they are contracted to provide to all their patients. This enhanced service specification outlines the more specialised services to be provided. The specification of this service is designed to cover enhanced aspects of clinical care of the patient with severe learning difficulties, which go beyond the scope of essential services. No part of the specification by commission, omission or implication defines or redefines essential or additional services.

This is a model local enhanced service (LES) for the provision of GMS for people with severe learning disabilities. Implementation should be considered in the context of the Assembly's Learning Disability Strategy Section 7 Guidance on Service Principles and Service Responses issued in August 2004. This guidance emphasises the need for joint working and partnership planning. It makes the point that one of the keys to success is joint working between local authorities, the NHS, voluntary bodies, users and carers. One of the service principles set out in the guidance is that people with learning disabilities have an equal right of access to primary healthcare services. The corresponding service response is to point to LESs under the GMS contract as one way of addressing these health needs. This model LES is intended to assist local partnerships to use enhanced services to deliver better healthcare to patients with learning disabilities.

Background

Evidence shows that:
- A GMS doctor with a list of 2000 patients will have about eight patients with severe learning disabilities
- People with learning disabilities, as a group, have much greater health needs than the general population. They are more likely to have general health problems, sensory impairments, mental health problems, epilepsy, cerebral palsy and other physical disabilities
- The uptake of breast and cervical screening by women with learning disabilities is poor
- People with learning disabilities tend to access primary care much less than they need to
- Many people with learning disabilities have undetected conditions that cause unnecessary suffering or reduce the quality or length of their lives.

All these patients are registered with a practice in Wales and therefore have access to a primary care team. The practice will have access to the medical record and history of these patients. Primary healthcare teams are well placed to assess the medical needs and monitor the health and well being of these patients.

Aims

The scheme will improve the quality of care provided through GMS to patients with learning disabilities. As a result it will enhance the life and independence of those patients. The scheme will achieve this by:

- Allowing practice teams to adopt a more proactive approach, spending more time with patients with learning disabilities and their carers so that any health problems are detected and treated at the earliest possible stage to minimise the risk to the patient's health
- Promoting a team-based approach to care, with improved liaison with carers, health and social care professionals.

The health check will constitute a 'specialist' assessment under the unified assessment process.

Service outline

Practices delivering the LES will be required to:

- Develop and maintain a register of those individuals who are on the local social services register for learning disabilities. This will include all patients with severe learning disabilities and, where applicable, their carers. This is to be used for audit purposes
- Demonstrate a systematic recall system for patients on the register
- Provide a health check, which will normally be on an annual basis. The health check will be based on the Welsh health check (attached), which is available on the Assembly GMS website and will be adapted for use with practice systems
- Integrate the health check as part of the patient's personal health record
- Involve carers and support workers. Where family or paid carers are involved, they can play a vital role in the patient's health care. With the consent of the patient, where possible, they should be fully informed of the patient's healthcare needs and supported as necessary
- Liaise with relevant local support services. Liaison with community and learning disability health professionals, social services and educational support services is necessary to provide seamless care for their patients and their carers. GPs should also, where appropriate, inform patients and their carers of local and national voluntary support groups for vital information and support.

All practices involved in the scheme will be required to conduct an annual review which will include:

- A review of the needs identified following completion of the health check and the outcome of the actions that were identified in order to meet these needs
- A brief report on feedback from patients and carers.

Professional quality assurance

Members of the primary healthcare team who are involved with providing this service should be in a position to demonstrate through their continuing professional development and appraisal that they have the necessary experience, training and competence to provide this service effectively.

Costs

For negotiation.

Welsh health check for people with a learning disability

Date:……………….………………… Name:……………….…………………..

Marital status:……………….………. Ethnic origin:…………………..……… …

Principal carer:…………………..……….

Date of birth:…………………..…………Sex: ……………….…………………..

Address:

………………………………………………………………………………………

………………………………………………………………………………………

Tel:…………………………………

Weight (kg/stone):…………………….. Height (meters/feet): ……………………

Blood pressure:……………………… Urine analysis: ……………………………

Smoke (per day):……………………. Alcohol (units per week): ………………

Body mass index (weight in kg/height in m^2): …………………………………

Cholesterol/serum lipids: ………………………………………………………

Immunisation

People with learning disabilities should have the same regimes as others and the same contraindications apply.

Tetanus in last 10 years?	Yes ☐	No ☐
If no, has tetanus been given?	Yes ☐	No ☐
Has influenza vaccine been given?	Yes ☐	No ☐
Is hepatitis B status known?	Yes ☐	No ☐

Result? ………………………………………………………………………………

Cervical screen

People with learning disabilities have same indications for cervical cytology as others.

Is a smear indicated?	Yes ☐	No ☐

If yes, when was last smear? ……/……/……When is next due? ……/……/……

What was the result? …………………………………………………………

Mammography

This should be arranged as per local practice.

Has mammogram been performed? Yes ☐　　　　No ☐

Chronic illness

Does your patient suffer from any chronic illnesses?

Diabetes?　　　　　　　　Yes ☐　　　　No ☐

Asthma?　　　　　　　　　Yes ☐　　　　No ☐

SYSTEMS ENQUIRY

The answer to these will not always be available.

General

Respiratory cough?　　　　Yes ☐　　　　No ☐

Haemoptysis?　　　　　　Yes ☐　　　　No ☐

Sputum?　　　　　　　　　Yes ☐　　　　No ☐

Wheeze?　　　　　　　　　Yes ☐　　　　No ☐

Dyspnoea?　　　　　　　　Yes ☐　　　　No ☐

Cardiovascular system

Chest pain?　　　　　　　Yes ☐　　　　No ☐

Swelling of ankles?　　　　Yes ☐　　　　No ☐

Palpitations?　　　　　　　Yes ☐　　　　No ☐

Postural nocturnal dyspnoea?　Yes ☐　　　　No ☐

Cyanosis?　　　　　　　　Yes ☐　　　　No ☐

Abdomen

Constipation?　　　　　　Yes ☐　　　　No ☐

Weight loss?　　　　　　　Yes ☐　　　　No ☐

Diarrhoea?　　　　　　　　Yes ☐　　　　No ☐

Dyspepsia?	Yes ☐	No ☐
Melaena?	Yes ☐	No ☐
Rectal bleeding?	Yes ☐	No ☐
Faecal incontinence?	Yes ☐	No ☐
Feeding problems ?	Yes ☐	No ☐

Central nervous system
For epilepsy see later.

Faints?	Yes ☐	No ☐
Paraesthesia?	Yes ☐	No ☐
Weakness?	Yes ☐	No ☐

If yes, where? ....

Genitourinary system

Dysuria?	Yes ☐	No ☐
Frequency?	Yes ☐	No ☐
Haematuria?	Yes ☐	No ☐
Urinary incontinence?	Yes ☐	No ☐

If yes, has midstream urine been done? Yes ☐   No ☐

Would you consider other investigations? Yes ☐   No ☐

Gynaecological system

Dysmenorrhoea?	Yes ☐	No ☐
Intermenstrual bleeding?	Yes ☐	No ☐
Per vaginal discharge?	Yes ☐	No ☐
Is patient postmenopausal?	Yes ☐	No ☐
Contraceptives?	Yes ☐	No ☐

Other?..

Epilepsy

Does patient have epilepsy?   Yes ☐   No ☐

Type of fit ....

Frequency of seizures (fits/month) ..../..................

Over the last year have the fits

Worsened ☐   Remained the same ☐   Improved ☐

Anti-epileptic medication

Name	Dose/frequency	Levels (if indicated)
....	....	....
....	....	....
....	....	....

Side-effects observed in the patient:

....

....

....

Behavioural disturbance
Behavioural disturbance in people with a learning disability is often an indicator of other morbidity.

Aggression?   Yes ☐   No ☐

If yes, is this?   More than ☐   Less than ☐   Very ☐
                     once a month   once a month   infrequently

Self-injury?   Yes ☐   No ☐

If yes, is this?   More than ☐   Less than ☐   Very ☐
                     once a month   once a month   infrequently

Overactivity?   Yes ☐   No ☐

If yes, is this?   More than ☐   Less than ☐   Very ☐
                     once a month   once a month   infrequently

Other?

....

If yes, is this?   More than ☐   Less than ☐   Very ☐
                    once a month   once a month   infrequently

PHYSICAL EXAMINATION

General appearance

Anaemia?   Yes ☐   No ☐

Lymph nodes?   Yes ☐   No ☐

Clubbing?   Yes ☐   No ☐

Jaundice?   Yes ☐   No ☐

Hydration?   Yes ☐   No ☐

Cardiovascular system

Pulse: ....beats/minute   Blood pressure:......./.........mmHg

Heart sounds: ....   Shortness of breath: Yes ☐   No ☐

(describe) ....

Respiratory system

Respiratory rate: ....breaths/minute

Breath sounds?   Yes ☐   No ☐

Wheeze?   Yes ☐   No ☐

Tachypnoea?   Yes ☐   No ☐

Additional sounds? Yes ☐   No ☐

(describe) ....

Abdomen

Masses?   Yes ☐   No ☐

Liver?   Yes ☐   No ☐

Spleen?   Yes ☐   No ☐

Rectal examination indicated?   Yes ☐   No ☐

Results?

....

Central nervous system

It is often difficult and not relevant to perform a full neurological examination. However, people with a learning disability are particularly prone to abnormalities in vision, hearing and communication. A change in function would suggest further investigation is necessary.

Vision

Normal vision ☐   Minor visual problem ☐   Major visual problems ☐

Is the carer/key worker concerned?   Yes ☐   No ☐

When did the patient last see an optician?   ....../......../........

Is there a cataract?   Yes ☐   No ☐

Result of Snellen chart ....

Any other data ....

Hearing

Normal hearing ☐   Minor hearing problem ☐   Major hearing problem ☐

Is the carer/key worker concerned?   Yes ☐   No ☐

Does the patient wear a hearing aid?   Yes ☐   No ☐

Any wax?   Yes ☐   No ☐

Does the patient see an audiologist?   Yes ☐   No ☐

Other investigations

....

Communication

Does your patient communicate normally?   Yes ☐   No ☐

Does your patient communicate with aids?   Yes ☐   No ☐

Does your patient have a severe
communication problem?   Yes ☐   No ☐

Does your patient see a speech therapist?   Yes ☐   No ☐

Mobility

Is your patient fully mobile?   Yes ☐   No ☐

Is your patient fully mobile with aids?   Yes ☐   No ☐

Is your patient immobile?   Yes ☐   No ☐

Has immobility been assessed?   Yes ☐   No ☐

Dermatology

Any abnormality?   Yes ☐   No ☐

Diagnosis? ....

Breast

Any lumps?   Yes ☐   No ☐

Any discharge?   Yes ☐   No ☐

Nipple retraction?   Yes ☐   No ☐

Other investigations

Are any further investigations necessary?   Yes ☐   No ☐
If yes, please indicate ....

Syndrome-specific check

Certain syndromes causing learning disabilities are associated with increased
morbidity (information can be found in the education pack provided); for this
reason it is important to record the following.

Is the cause of learning disability known?   Yes ☐   No ☐

If yes, what is it? ....

Has the patient had a chromosomal analysis? Yes ☐   No ☐

Result? ....

What is the degree of learning disability?

Mild ☐   Moderate ☐   Severe ☐   Profound ☐

If your patient has Down's syndrome they should have a yearly test for hypothyroidism.

Has this been done?   Yes ☐   No ☐

Other medication

Drug	Dose	Side-effects	Levels (if indicated)
....	....	....	....
....	....	....	....
....	....	....	....
....	....	....	....
....	....	....	....

Thank you.

APPENDIX 17

POWYS LHB SPECIFICATION FOR A LOCAL ENHANCED SERVICE: TREATMENT ROOM PROCEDURES

Introduction

Historically, general medical practices have provided a range of services that fall outside those defined by the new GMS contract as being either essential or additional services.

These services have often been devolved to primary care from the providers of secondary or tertiary care. This local enhanced service encourages medical practices to continue providing these services for the benefit of patients. In doing so, patients will benefit from receiving their care locally, while reducing the workload of those working in secondary care.

Service outline

The range of services requested of medical practices is wide and varies between secondary care providers. However, the services provided *generally* fall within the following categories:

- Phlebotomy undertaken as part of a broader secondary care based service
- Pre-operative work-up undertaken as part of a broader secondary care based service
- Post-operative care undertaken as part of a broader secondary care based service
- Other procedures that are not part of essential, additional or any *current* enhanced service, but which in time may become subject to its own local enhanced service.

To qualify for payment under this local enhanced service, medical practices must confirm they are involved, where currently requested, in all four areas of activity.

Medical practice requirements

A medical practice providing these services must have:

- Satisfactory facilities
- Appropriate nursing and/or healthcare assistant support
- Sterilisation and infection control procedures to a standard acceptable to the LHB
- A system to ensure that appropriate informed consent is obtained and recorded
- A system, acceptable to the LHB, for recording and sending of specimens and receiving laboratory reports
- A system, acceptable to the LHB, enabling the auditing of procedures undertaken and the monitoring of clinical outcomes.

Accreditation

Doctors, nurses, healthcare assistants and other healthcare professionals will provide these services in accordance with their own personal identified competencies. Each will need to have undertaken appropriate training and work within their professional/personal competencies and undertake annual appraisal.

Pricing

Payment for the provision of this local enhanced service will be made on the basis of a fee per registered patient. The payment will be Xp per patient registered with the medical practice as at 1 April 2004.

APPENDIX 18

DYFED POWYS LMC SPECIFICATION FOR A LOCAL ENHANCED SERVICE: MINOR INJURY SERVICES

Introduction

All practices are expected to provide essential and those additional services they are contracted to provide to all their patients. This enhanced service specification for the provision of minor injury services outlines the more specialised services to be provided. The specification of this service is designed to cover the enhanced aspects of clinical care of the patient, all of which are beyond the scope of essential services. No part of the specification by commission, omission or implication defines or redefines essential or additional services.

This specification sets out an in-hours service. It is therefore a requirement of the scheme that the participating medical practice is available to readily provide a minor injuries service between the hours of 8.00am and 6.30pm every week day (bank and public holidays excluded).

Background

This NES recognises the need for a consistent approach to rewarding GPs equitably for providing minor injury services within their own practice. This service will be commissioned in the context of reforming emergency care services and reducing pressure on accident and emergency departments and hospital-based minor injuries units.

Outside the conurbations and those towns having a district general hospital based accident and emergency service, local GPs for historical and professional ethical reasons have had to provide minor injury services either at their surgery premises or in a minor injury unit, usually attached to a community hospital.

Professional consensus indicates that injuries and wounds over 48 hours old should usually be dealt with through normal primary care services as should any lesion of a non-traumatic origin. By definition, such cases are usually the self-presenting 'walking wounded' and ambulance cases are not usually accepted except by individual prior agreement between the doctor and the attending ambulance personnel.

The following list gives guidance on the types of injuries and circumstances that lead to the use of minor injury services. **It is not intended to be a comprehensive list.**

- Lacerations capable of closure by simple techniques (stripping, gluing, suturing)
- Bruises

- Minor dislocations of phalanges
- Foreign bodies
- Non-penetrating superficial ocular foreign bodies
- Following advice to attend specifically given by a GP
- Following recent injury of a severity not amenable to simple domestic first aid
- Following recent injury where it is suspected stitches may be required
- Following blows to the head where there has been no loss of consciousness
- Recent eye injury
- Partial thickness thermal burns or scalds involving broken skin:
  (a) Not over 1 inch diameter
  (b) Not involving the hands, feet, face, neck, genital areas
- Foreign bodies superficially embedded in tissues
- Minor trauma to hands, limbs or feet.

Service outline
This national enhanced service will fund:
- Initial triage including immediately necessary clinical action to staunch haemorrhage and prevent further exacerbation of the injury
- History taking, relevant clinical examination and documentation
- Wound assessment to ascertain suitability for locally based treatment and immediate wound dressing and toilet where indicated
- Appropriate and timely referral and/or follow-up arrangements
- Adequate facilities including premises and equipment, as are necessary to enable the proper provision of minor injury services including facilities for cardiopulmonary resuscitation
- Registered nurses to provide care and support to patients undergoing minor injury services
- Maintenance of infection control standards
- Information to patients on the treatment options and the treatment proposed. The patient should give written consent for the procedure to be carried out and the completed consent form should be filed in the patient's lifelong medical record
- Transmission of all tissue removed by minor surgery for histological examination where appropriate
- Maintenance of records of all procedures
- Audit of minor surgery list work at regular intervals. This audit should include an element of peer review by conducting it in collaboration with a local specialist or GP colleague working in the same field or with audit groups. Reviews of this work could examine patient satisfaction and compare preoperative diagnosis with the histology reports where relevant. Any complications arising from the surgical procedure should be recorded. Other suitable topics for audit include clinical outcomes, rates of infection and unexpected or incomplete excision of basal cell tumours or malignant pigmented lesions.

Patients in the following categories are not appropriate for treatment by the minor injury service, but the enhanced service covers the appropriate referral of these patients elsewhere. **This list is for guidance only. Clinicians should practise within their individual competencies.**

- 999 call (unless attending crew speak directly to the doctor)
- Any patient who cannot be discharged home after treatment
- Any patient with airway, breathing, circulatory or neurological compromise
- Actual or suspected overdose
- Accidental ingestion, poisoning, fume or smoke inhalation
- Blows to the head with loss of consciousness or extremes of age
- Sudden collapse or fall in a public place
- Penetrating eye injury
- Chemical, biological, or radioactive contamination injured patients
- Full thickness burns
- Burns caused by electric shock
- Partial thickness burns over 3 cm diameter or involving:
  - Injuries to organs of special sense
  - Injuries to the face, neck, hands, feet or genitalia
- New or unexpected bleeding from any body orifice if profuse
- Foreign bodies impacted in bodily orifices, especially in children
- Foreign bodies deeply embedded in tissues
- Trauma to hands, limbs or feet substantially affecting function
- Penetrating injuries to the head, torso, abdomen
- Lacerating/penetrating injuries involving nerve, artery or tendon damage.

Child protection arrangements
Each medical practice will ensure it has access to:
- All Wales Child Protection procedures and related child protection policies/protocols and guidelines.
- *Working Together to Safeguard Children*, 2000
- Social services child protection phone numbers
- Contact details of LHB 'named' nurses and doctors
- Contact details for paediatric advice
- A system to notify the health visitor/school nurse of all <16 child attendances
- A nominated lead GP for child protection.

For each child attendance, the medical practice will record:
- Date and time of attendance
- Full name (including any other surname in use), address, date of birth and telephone number
- Name of parent or primary carer
- Person with 'parental responsibility' (including who is giving consent) if under 16
- Name and details of person accompanying, if not above
- Details of 'care' status (i.e. any known legal orders in place).

The medical practice must always be vigilant in the history taking and examination of children and be prepared to consider child abuse as a possible cause in all presentations. The medical practice will note that young children, especially those under the age of 2 years, are more likely to be seriously injured or killed.

GPs involved in this scheme must be familiar with the child protection process and ensure they receive child protection training to at least levels 1 and 2.

Child protection referral

Staff involved in the delivery of this scheme must be aware of how to make a child protection referral to the social services department. It is the responsibility of the attending GP to make the referral. Any child protection referral by telephone must be followed up in writing within 48 hours.

GPs must be aware that where there are child protection issues, even if the police are already involved, a child protection referral should still be made to the social services department. GPs must be fully aware of when and how to check the child protection register.

Child protection: good practice guidelines

Presentations to cause concern (always consider further advice)

- Frequent attender
- Inconsistent and/or changing history
- Examination and explanation not compatible
- Delay in presentation
- Concern about parental interaction
- Concern about parenting capacity
- Domestic abuse
- Alcohol/substance misuse
- Self-harm
- Signs of neglect

Injuries to cause concern (must seek further advice)

- Any bruise/injury (however minor) in a baby under 6 months or to any non-ambulant child
- Any severe bruising/fracture/head injury in a child under 1 year or in any child not walking
- Injuries/bruises caused by implements
- Bruises to the face/ears/inner surfaces of limbs/genitalia
- Bruising that is excessive
- Scalds/cigarette burns
- Certain fractures of ribs/long bones/metaphyseal/skull in a young child

Concern identified	Action
• Where there are obvious child protection concerns	• Make a child protection referral to the social services department
• Where there are obvious child protection concerns and the child is also admitted	• Make a child protection referral and agree this with paediatrics department
• Where there are issues and injuries of concern (see above)	• Always seek paediatric advice from a senior paediatrician
• Where advice is needed about the child protection procedures	• Seek advice as above or from the LHB named professionals
• If the child is removed from the practice premises and there are child protection concerns	• Contact social services department immediately and, if necessary, the police
• You have considered making an enquiry to the child protection register	• Make a formal enquiry of the social services department child protection register

For all of the above it is also helpful to discuss with the named doctor/nurse.

Where a child protection referral is made:

- A phone referral to the social services department must be followed up with a written referral within two days
- The LHB named nurse should be informed
- The patient's GP, health visitor and school nurse should be informed as soon as possible and within one working day.

Data recording arrangements

In the longer term, medical practices will be required to enter clinical data in the LHB MIP system. Initially, medical practices are required to collect and retain data in accordance with the LHB minor injury unit clinical record. Wherever possible, a template in accordance with the parameters of this record should be established on the medical practice's own clinical system.

Facilities and equipment requirements

In terms of treatment room fittings, the following **must** be provided by the medical practice:

- Room no less than 17.5m² in size, fitted with adequate units (some lockable), with work surfaces
- Dedicated drug fridge
- Adequate treatment couch
- Good-quality overhead examination lamp
- Hand basin with elbow taps, soap dispenser and alcohol gel
- Paper towel dispenser
- Oxygen source.

Instruments used must either be single use, disposable instruments or appropriately cleaned and sterilised reusables. The medical practice should have available appropriate equipment to deal with minor injuries. The medical practice should hold in stock an appropriate range and quantity of consumables to deal with minor injuries.

Service availability and response times

The service must be available between the hours of 8.00am and 6.30pm weekdays (excluding bank and public holidays). The service must be available to all patients requiring treatment for a minor injury. The service must be equally available to both those who are and who are not patients registered with the practice for GMS purposes.

A patient arriving at the practice during the hours of 9.00am to 5.00pm and in need of treatment for a minor injury must be assessed by a suitably qualified doctor or nurse within 15 minutes of their arrival. During the hours of 8.00am and 9.00am and 5.00pm and 6.30pm, this assessment must take place within 30 minutes.

Service provider accreditation

Doctors providing minor injury services would be expected to have:

- Current experience of provision of minor injury work or
- Current minor surgery experience or
- Recent accident and emergency experience or
- Equivalent training that satisfies relevant appraisal and revalidation procedures.

Doctors carrying out minor injury services must be competent in resuscitation and, as for other areas of clinical practice, have a responsibility for ensuring that their skills are regularly updated. Doctors carrying out minor injury activity should demonstrate a continuing sustained level of activity, conduct audit data and take part in appropriate educational activities.

Nurses assisting in minor injury procedures should be appropriately trained and competent taking into consideration their professional accountability and the Nursing and Midwifery Council guidelines on the scope of professional practice.

Those doctors who have previously provided services similar to the proposed enhanced service and who satisfy at appraisal and revalidation that they have such continuing medical experience, training and competence as is necessary to enable them to contract for the enhanced service shall be deemed professionally qualified to do so.

Pricing

Prices associated with this scheme are set up in Annex A attached [note: this is not included here].

Infection control arrangements

The importance of infection control

Hospital-acquired infection occurs in approximately 10% of patients in acute hospitals. Factors such as underlying disease, surgery and immunosuppressive therapies make hospitalised patients more susceptible to infection than the general population. In addition, they may be exposed to infection through contact with other infected patients. The most common infections are those of the urinary tract, surgical wounds and the lower respiratory tract. Other problems include infections at intravenous catheter sites.

The emergence of antibiotic resistant organisms such as methicillin resistant *Staphylococcus aureus* is a particular problem in hospitals.

Infections cause the patient pain and discomfort, add to their length of stay in hospital and are a major cause of morbidity and mortality. Increased length of hospitalisation due to infection is costly and has an adverse effect on waiting lists. The cost of antibiotics, dressings and investigations is considerable.

Not all hospital-acquired infection can be prevented due to the vulnerability of hospitalised patients, but good infection control practices can reduce the risk of avoidable infection and cross infection.

Principles of infection control

It is important that all staff working in medical practices understand the principles used in preventing the spread of infection, and apply them to their everyday working practices. Prevention of infection is the responsibility of *all* healthcare workers.

For any infection to develop in a patient three things must happen. This is known as the 'chain of infection'. First, there must be a source of infectious organisms. In practice, most sources are other patients suffering from infection or colonised by a microorganism. Occasionally, the source is an inanimate object or the physical environment where the patient is being treated. However, these are less important.

Even when a source of infection is present, the infection may not spread to other patients unless it is transmitted to them in some way. Transmission is the second link in the chain of infection; there are several ways by which infection may be spread:

- **Direct contact** – this involves the direct physical transfer of organisms through personal contact with a source and other patients. This is usually via the hands of medical and nursing staff. It is by far the most important way by which infection is spread and is the reason why so much emphasis is placed on hand washing

- **Indirect contact** – the microorganisms are transferred between a source and other patients by contaminated objects, e.g. improperly decontaminated instruments, respiratory equipment, commodes, beds, etc

- **Airborne transmission** – organisms can be transmitted by droplets from people with infections affecting the respiratory tract (e.g. tuberculosis) or by dust and skin scales (e.g. in staphylococcus infections)

- **Blood and body fluids** – these are potentially hazardous because infections such as hepatitis and HIV can be transmitted through inoculation injury, breaks in the skin, gross contamination of mucous membranes, sexual activity or pre-natally from mother to baby

- **Food-borne transmission** – infections are caused when contaminated food is ingested (e.g. salmonella infection)

- **Vector-borne transmission** – some insects carry pathogenic organisms on their bodies and in their digestive tracts; this may infect the hospital environment, which includes food and sterile supplies. It is essential that supplies are stored in dry, clean and well-ventilated areas to prevent infestation.

The third link in the chain is a susceptible host. Unfortunately, by their nature, hospitals are full of susceptible hosts. It is important to remember that ill people are much more susceptible to infection than those who are well. Certain factors compound this, such as surgery, trauma, radiotherapy and immunosuppression, producing a patient who is very vulnerable to infection.

From time to time updated advice on cross infection control and, for example, the decontamination and sterilisation of surgical instruments, is published by the Welsh Assembly Government. Medical practices should be aware of and implement the most recent guidance that has been made available.

Preventing the spread of infection
This involves nothing more than interrupting the links in the chain of infection. This is achieved by a combination of following the principles of standard (universal) precautions and infection control principles, which include:
- Effective hand washing or clean hand disinfection before any procedure
- Wearing personal protective clothing for any clinical/invasive procedure
- Safe disposal of clinical waste
- Safe disposal of sharps

- Safe disposal of linen that is soiled/contaminated/infected
- Safe disposal of blood and body fluid spillages, using the correct procedure at all times
- Covering all skin lesions with a waterproof dressing
- Proper decontamination and sterilisation of all reusable equipment used on patients
- Where possible, encouraging use of single use medical devices
- Barrier nursing of patients that require it
- Ensuring the clinical environment is adequately cleaned regularly
- Ensuring food hygiene standards are maintained.

All medical practices providing a minor injuries service are advised to have a copy of the Powys Local Health Board Infection Control Policy folder.

It is the responsibility of *all* medical and nursing staff to ensure they have annual training in infection control and are aware of the following infection control policies:
- Standard (universal) precautions
- Inoculation injury policy
- Hand wash/hand decontamination policy
- Handling of blood and body fluids
- Collection of specimens
- Decontamination policy.

APPENDIX 19

BRIGHTON AND HOVE PCT SPECIFICATION FOR A LOCAL ENHANCED SERVICE: DIAGNOSING AND TREATING MAJOR DEPRESSION

Background

This local enhanced service (LES) recognises the high demand placed on primary care by patients with depression in Brighton and Hove. In conjunction with practice counsellors, the new primary care mental health workers and the alcohol and drugs misuse enhanced services, the aim of this LES is to improve the quality of care provided to patients with depression in primary care. The specification of this service is designed to cover the enhanced aspects of clinical care of the patient that are beyond the scope of essential services.

Service outline

Depression is the second most common cause of disability worldwide and the third most common reason for consultation in general practice. While depression is common, it is often missed in primary care and this is particularly true of patients presenting with non-specific physical symptoms. Using the DMS-IV diagnostic criteria,[1] depression can be divided into three main groups according to number and duration of symptoms (Table 1):

- Minor depression
- Major depression (which is further divided into mild, moderate and severe)
- Dysthymia.

Table 1. Diagnostic categories for depression and dysthymia and suggested first-line treatments

Diagnostic category	Number of symptoms	Duration	Suggested first-line treatment
Minor depression	2–4 depressive symptoms, including depressed mood or anhedonia	2 weeks	Support, counselling, sleep management, problem solving
Major depression	*Mild*: 5 symptoms, minor impact on ability to cope with life/work *Moderate*: 6+ symptoms, major impact on life/work *Severe*: 6–7+ symptoms of increased severity with marked impact on life/work	2 weeks	*Mild*: as for minor with structured follow up *Moderate* or *severe*: antidepressants/cognitive behaviour therapy/ referral to community mental health team/psychology

Dysthymia	3 or 4 depressive symptoms including depressed mood	2 years	Antidepressants

See Panel 1 for details of symptoms.

Unrecognised **major** depression is associated with poor treatment outcomes and it is therefore important to identify this group and then offer effective interventions and treatments. For moderate and severe major depression (see Table 1 and Panel 1 for definitions) this will usually involve prescribing an antidepressant and providing structured follow up and referral to more specialised services when necessary and according to patient choice. Antidepressants need to be used in adequate doses and for at least four to six months following remission (see *British National Formulary* and local guidelines).

Milder forms of depression are also very common. These can be called **minor** depression if not meeting the criteria for major depression and **mild** depression if just meeting the criteria (see Table 1 and Panel 1). They will often resolve spontaneously over time,[2] and the challenge for primary care is to accurately diagnose this group of patients and then offer appropriate interventions. The evidence for the use of antidepressants in this group of patients is weak and other interventions (such as problem solving, counselling, sleep management, exercise advice) are usually more appropriate. Some patients will become more severely depressed and structured follow up is therefore important so as to be able to respond to changing patient needs over time.

Dysthymia is defined by the presence of at least three symptoms, including depressed mood, on more days than not for at least two years. There is evidence that antidepressants are useful for this group of patients.

Depression often becomes a relapsing and chronic condition and interventions need to be designed to improve care over the long term. This may require sustained or repeated treatment and will need a structured approach similar to that used in the management of other chronic conditions such as asthma and diabetes.

The training of GPs and practice staff and the development of guidelines and protocols improve skills but do not necessarily improve outcomes for patients.[3] However, multifaceted interventions (case management by practice nurses, clinician education, greater integration with secondary care) can improve outcomes in depression. The use of telephone follow up has been shown to be a simple intervention that improves the care and outcome of depression.[4]

The management of depression in primary care therefore involves many stages and forms the basis of the Brighton and Hove LES for depression, as follows:
- Identifying people with dysthymia and major depression and rating the severity of major depression as mild, moderate or severe (see Table 1 and Panel 1)
- Producing and maintaining a practice-based register of these patients (see below)
- Managing the majority of patients with mild depression with non-drug interventions
- Managing patients with moderate and severe major depression or dysthymia with antidepressants at adequate drug dosages and referring to more specialised services when necessary, available and according to patient choice

- Using locally developed protocols to guide patient assessment and management
- Provide structured follow up for patients, which might include telephone follow up by nurses
- Regular audit of outcome measures
- Undertaking training (if needed) in the assessment and management of depression (to be provided by Brighton and Hove PCT).

Setting up the register
- Search for patients already coded for depression. For 5 byte there are many different codes for depression, but most will probably be picked up by searching under the following Read code groups:
  - Eu32%   [X] Depressive episode
  - Eu33%   [X] Recurrent depressive episode
  - Eu341   [X] Dysthymia
  - E2003   Anxiety with depression
  - E204   Postnatal depression
  - E2B%   Depression NEC
  - 1BT   Depressed mood

- Search for patients on common antidepressant drugs with none of the above codes.

- Try to assign one of the following codes to each patient:
  - Eu320   [X] Mild depressive episode
  - Eu321   [X] Moderated depressive episode
  - Eu323   [X] Severe depressive episode, no psychotic symptoms
  - Eu324   [X] Severe depressive episode, with psychotic symptoms
  - Eu33%   [X] Recurrent depressive disorder (see subcodes for severity)
  - Eu341   [X] Dysthymia
  - 1BT   Depressed mood
              (if not meeting the criteria for major depression)

If the severity of the episode is not known, use *Eu32 [X] depressive episode* until a more accurate diagnosis is made. If other codes for depression (such as the older E2... codes) are routinely used in the practice then clinicians may wish to continue using them but should be aware that the severity of depression is not easy to code.

Audit and verification
The following audit will need to be performed annually and data collection sheets will be sent to participating practices (Table 2). The percentages are suggested targets only (payments will *not* depend on reaching these targets).

Table 2. Criteria and suggested targets for audit

Criteria	Target
1. Up-to-date register of patients with major depression	
2. Percentage of patients with major depression in whom the severity of the depression is recorded as mild, moderate or severe	70%

3. Percentage of patients with major depression who have
   had their suicide risk assessed   90%

4. Percentage of patients with moderate or severe major
   depression who have been treated with antidepressants
   or referred for psychological therapy according to
   patient choice   90%

5. Percentage of patients treated with full dose
   antidepressants for six months or more unless not
   tolerated or ineffective*   90%

6. Percentage of patients who have had a review
   appointment within one month of starting medication*   90%

*These criteria may not be easy to audit electronically due to current lack of
appropriate Read codes. If a notes search is required a random sample of 30% of
patients on the register may be selected for a notes review. This advice may be
amended as new codes and national guidance emerge.

See Panel 2 for a suggested computer template and Read codes for data collection.

Costs

Practices participating in this LES will receive 35p per registered patient (list size
as at 1 April 2004). This will be paid as follows:
- 50% in 12 monthly payments (backdated to April 2004) to reflect the work
  associated with setting up registers and templates, adopting a management
  protocol based on the information supplied in this document and providing the
  enhanced services for the remainder of the year
- 50% for completing the audit associated with depression at the end of the year,
  which will be supplied by the PCT.

As prevalence data are gathered from practices, these payments may alter to
reflect the increased workload involved for practices with a large number of
patients on the register.

References

1. American Psychiatric Association. *Diagnostic and Statistical Manual of Mental
   Disorders*. Fourth edition. Washington: American Psychiatric Association,
   1994.
2. Simon GE *et al*. Outcome of recognized and unrecognized depression in an
   international primary care study. *Gen Hosp Psychiatry* 1999;21:97–105.
3. Gilbody SM *et al*. Routinely administered questionnaires for depression and
   anxiety: systematic review. *BMJ* 2001;322:406–9.
4. Improving the recognition and management of depression in primary care.
   Effective Health Care Bulletin 2002;7(No. 5).

Panel 1: **Diagnosing depression in primary care**

Screen for patients using two questions:
- During the last month, have you often been bothered by feeling down, depressed or hopeless?
- During the last month, have you often been bothered by feeling little interest or pleasure in doing things?

Increase the accuracy of the diagnosis by using the DSM-IV diagnostic criteria for depression. A major depressive illness exists if the patient has a low mood or loss of pleasure or interest for at least two weeks and a positive score on at least five of the following:
- Abnormal depressed mood
- Anhedonia (marked loss of pleasure or interest)
- Sleep disturbance
- Appetite or weight disturbance
- Disturbance in activity (agitation or slowing)
- Fatigue or loss of energy
- Guilt or feelings of worthlessness
- Impaired concentration
- Thoughts of suicide.

Fewer than five symptoms can be called minor depression.

Major depression can be classified as mild, moderate or severe, as follows:
- **Mild depression** – five symptoms, little impact on ability to socialise or work
- **Moderate depression** – six or more symptoms with significant impact on ability to work or socialise
- **Severe depression** – seven or more symptoms, including symptoms of increased severity such as agitation or suicidal thoughts and major impact on life or work

A patient can be diagnosed as having **dysthymia** if they have three or four depressive symptoms, including depressed mood, for two years.

The ICD-10 criteria for the diagnosis of depression and definitions of severity are very similar. The use of screening questionnaires (such as the Beck's inventory) can be useful in increasing detection in patients if the clinician suspects depression and can be useful in monitoring progress. Their use has not been shown to improve clinical outcomes.

Panel 2: **Example template for managing depression with Read codes (5 byte)**

Prompt	Pick-list with Read codes	
Initial assessment	6653	Y/N
Follow-up psychiatric assessment	6654	Y/N
Depressed mood?	Normal mood	1BS0
	Depressed mood	1BT
Loss of interest?	No loss of interest	1BS1
	Loss of interest	1BP
Duration in weeks?		Text box
Sleep disturbance?	Good sleep pattern	1B1R
	Delayed-onset sleep	1BX0
	Excessive sleep	1BX1
	Early morning waking	1BX3
Appetite disturbance?	Normal appetite	1611
	Loss of appetite	1612
	Increased appetite	1613
Activity levels?	Agitation	1B16
	Psychomotor retardation	1P01
Fatigue?	No fatigue	1681
	Fatigue	1682
Guilt?	No guilt	1BS3
	Guilty ideas	1BF
Impaired concentration?	Normal concentration	1BS2
	Impaired concentration	1BR
Suicidal thoughts? (1B19)	High suicide risk	1BD5
	Moderate suicide risk	1BD6
	Low suicide risk	1BD7
Depression score	Minor depression <5 symptoms	
	Major depression 5+ symptoms	
	• Mild: 5 symptoms	
	• Moderate: 6+ symptoms	
	• Severe: 7+ symptoms,	
	Dysthymia; low mood >2 years	
Mental state diagnosis	Depressed (minor)	IB17
	Mild depressive episode	Eu320
	Moderate depressive episode	Eu321
	Severe depressive episode without psychotic symptoms	Eu322
	Severe depressive episode with psychotic symptoms	Eu323

	Recurrent depressive disorder, current episode mild	Eu330
	Recurrent depressive disorder, current episode moderate	Eu331
	Recurrent depressive episode, current episode severe, no psychosis	Eu332
	Recurrent depressive disorder, current episode severe, psychotic symptoms	Eu333
	Dysthymia	Eu341
Psychiatric treatment started	6659	Y/N
Psychiatric treatment stopped	665A	Y/N
Adverse reaction to antidepressants	TJ90	Y/N
Psychiatric drugs side-effects	6655	Y/N
Driving advice	8CAJ	Y/N
Treatment options	Self-help literature	8CE
	Sleep management	8Q0
	Exercise advice	8CA5
	Problem solving	8G96
Referral?	Referred to counsellor	8H78
	Referred to gateway worker	8H7A
	Referred to community mental health team	8H7B
	Referred to psychologist (cognitive behaviour therapy)	8H7T
	Referred to psychiatrist	8H49
Follow up	8H8	Prompt for date

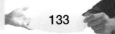

INDEX